MEDICINE
FROM THE
KITCHEN

"With a wealth of experience from decades of alopathic nursing, herbology and refined earth-wisdom Jesse Emerson RN has compiled a wonderful guide full of common-sense, insightful remedies to navigate the course of many conditions and maladies. She invokes the advice of Western medicinal approaches with an eye to folk-medicine, traditional cures and her own time-tested concoctions. This little edition* offers a simple way to treat many emergency situations and awakens the reader to solutions that may be staring us in the face when we open our minds and our cabinets to the healing power of common occupants: spices, herbs, teas, fruits, vegetables, and unusual liniments. In an age when we are bombarded with the insistence of pharmaceuticals into our lives, it is refreshing to be reminded of ways to address healing that are low-tech, surprisingly sensible, AND accessible in the treasure trove of Nature's own pantry and pharmacy."

-**Seth Mark Friedman**, D.C.
Santa Fe, NM

MEDICINE FROM THE KITCHEN

*Safe and Simple Remedies from the Kitchen
for First Aid and Minor Ailments*

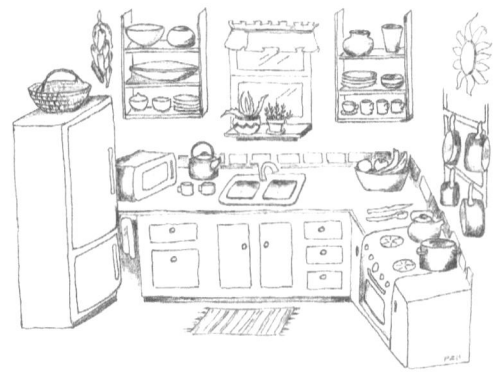

"Leave your drugs in the chemist's pot if
you can heal the patient with food."
Hippocrates

BE PREPARED FOR ANY EMERGENCY
READ THIS BOOK NOW

Jessie L. Emerson RN, Certified Clinical Herbalist

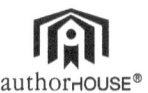

AuthorHouse™ LLC
1663 Liberty Drive
Bloomington, IN 47403
www.authorhouse.com
Phone: 1-800-839-8640

© 2014 Jessie L. Emerson. All rights reserved.

No part of this book may be reproduced, stored in a retrieval system, or transmitted by any means without the written permission of the author.

Published by AuthorHouse   08/23/2014

ISBN: 978-1-4969-0576-5 (sc)
ISBN: 978-1-4969-0577-2 (e)

Library of Congress Control Number: 2014907264

Any people depicted in stock imagery provided by Thinkstock are models, and such images are being used for illustrative purposes only. Certain stock imagery © Thinkstock.

This book is printed on acid-free paper.

Because of the dynamic nature of the Internet, any web addresses or links contained in this book may have changed since publication and may no longer be valid. The views expressed in this work are solely those of the author and do not necessarily reflect the views of the publisher, and the publisher hereby disclaims any responsibility for them.

The purpose of this booklet is to provide basic information on first aid for some of the most common injuries and illnesses.

REMEMBER:

If symptoms persist or become more severe: SEEK PROFESSIONAL HELP IMMEDIATELY. The author and publisher disclaim any responsibility or liability for any loss that may occur as a result of the information, procedures, or techniques presented.

TABLE OF CONTENTS

1. SAFETY RULES WHEN USING HOME REMEDIES 1
2. AILMENTS, EMERGENCIES, AND REMEDIES 3
3. TIPS ON HOW TO DO IT 40
4. MY FAVORITE TEAS TO KEEP IN THE KITCHEN 46
5. TEA TIPS 50
6. LIST OF SPICES—MEDICINAL USES 52
7. RECIPIES..59
8. APPENDICES 63
   A. GLOSSARY 63
   B. KITCHEN EQUIPMENT 68
   C. OTHER KITCHEN NECESSITIES...............................70
   D. U.S. AND METRIC MEASURES 76
   E. BASIC FIRST AID KITS 77
   F. RESOURCES AND REFERENCES...............................79
   G. FAMILY MEDICAL INFORMATION 80

I dedicate this little booklet to all those who desire to be self-sufficient and sustainable. I believe being prepared, awake, and aware is your best insurance.

A special thanks to Phoebe Hummel for her wonderful drawings and to Jared Gann for his help in preparing the manuscript.

INTRODUCTION

This little handbook is my personal collection of tried and true first aid remedies. Some are folk remedies from different cultures that have worked for me, some I learned from my wonderful teacher, Michael Moore, some are from friends and some originate from using them and seeing what works and what doesn't. Although there are many herbal remedies, this booklet focuses on what can be found in the kitchen, with the addition of a few common herbs that are easily obtained.

Kitchens contain many simple, yet effective, first aid remedies. They are based on the Western Herbal Medicine tradition.

It is my belief that we must know what to do when there is no doctor or what to do until medical help is available. I have been personally empowered by my knowledge of herbs, and being able to confidently treat minor ailments and medical emergencies. Those who read this book will learn safe and effective treatments. I am excited to share this knowledge with you, so you too may become empowered in this arena and that you will be inspired to equip your kitchen with the herbs, spices, foods, and other remedies, which will be helpful in times of medical need.

Do not wait until an emergency to read this book. Prevention, knowledge, and staying calm in a crisis are the three necessary ingredients in a safe and healthful life.

Have fun, be safe, and know what to do if . . .

Jessie Emerson

SAFETY RULES WHEN USING HOME REMEDIES

1. Stay calm.
2. Knowing what to do before the emergency helps you stay calm.
3. Learn CPR and the Heimlich maneuver, and take a First Aid course.
4. Evaluate the whole person, situation, and circumstances.
5. Know when to seek professional help.
6. Know what to do until there is professional help.
7. Use the information in this book as directed.
8. If you try a remedy and it does not work, try another remedy; and depending on the circumstances, you may need professional help.
9. Diabetics with foot injuries should see a health care professional immediately. Do not try to self-help in this circumstance.
10. Monitor your progress. After a few days, reevaluate.
11. Stop treatment if there is any adverse reactions or if the treatment is not helping.
12. Record keeping: Keep notes of remedies used and the outcomes, especially any adverse reactions. Keep a concise medical record on yourself and family members. List the medications each person takes on a daily basis. Note any medication and food allergies and the reactions to them.
13. When in doubt, SEEK PROFESSIONAL HELP.

PREVENTION IS THE KEY FOR EMERGENCY SITUATIONS

- Poison proof your home.
- Know what plants are poisonous and unsafe for children and pets.
- Learn the venomous creatures where you live, what they look like, their natural habitat, and the sign and symptoms of their bite.
- Have an emergency plan for fire, flood, etc. and practice it.

- ❖ Have a fire extinguisher in your home and car.
- ❖ Basic first aid kits for home, car, and backpack. A good first aide book is a must.

BE AWARE, BE ALERT, BE PREPARED

AILMENTS, EMERGENCIES, AND REMEDIES

The first rule of first aid: WASH YOUR HANDS BEFORE AND AFTER WORKING WITH A PERSON. Wear gloves. Wash hands before putting on gloves and after removing them. Dispose of them in an appropriate manner.

First aid Guidelines:

1. Prompt rescue for safety reasons: e.g. removing from water, fire, smoke, and carbon monoxide.
2. Make sure the victim has an open airway.
3. Control bleeding.
4. Give first aid for poisoning.
5. Always keep a list of emergency phone numbers available.
6. Assess for and treat medical problems that are not life threatening.
7. When immediate problems are under control:

    A. Find out exactly what happened.
    B. Look for emergency medical information.

8. Know your capabilities; know when to seek medical help.

ANXIETY or NERVOUSNESS:

1. Rosemary tea
2. Lavender tea, apply lavender oil to temples, smell oil
3. Celery seed tea
4. Vinegar compresses to forehead and body for nighttime restlessness, especially with the flu
5. Hot baths: add ginger or rosemary tea, Epsom salts
6. Bee pollen daily: start with ¼ tsp. and gradually work up to 1 tsp. daily (or vitamin B complex, as directed). Do not take if allergic to bee pollen.

ASTHMA:

Eliminate cow's milk from diet, use goat milk products, and eliminate white flour and sugar from diet; could be a reaction to chlorine used to bleach the flour and sugar.

Acute episodes: Have person lightly bite the back of their tongue.

1. Coffee, very strong, 2-3 cups, espresso (this may not work if the person is already a heavy caffeine user).
2. Make hot chocolate according to directions.
3. 1 ½ oz. of dark chocolate bar, repeat until relief
4. Thyme tea: (expectorant and bronchial dilator), 1 cup every hour until relief.
5. Teas: Anise, fennel, cardamom, marjoram, 1 cup every 1-2 hours as needed.
6. Green tea: anti-inflammatory, 1 cup 2 times a day and as needed. (This works if you are not a regular tea drinker.)

ATHLETES' FOOT AND OTHER FUNGAL INFECTIONS:

Fungal infections: most fungal infections grow in a circle and often itch. On the head there is often loss of hair. Fingernails and toenails become rough and thick. Often washing the infected part with soap and water two times a day is all that is needed. Keep the affected part dry, change socks and underwear often. Expose feet to sunlight daily.

1. Make a tea with garlic cloves: mash 3-6 cloves, pour 1 cup hot water over it and steep (let soak) 15-20 minutes. Pour into a warm foot bath, soak 15-20 minutes, do this nightly.
2. Licorice: (use real licorice not the candy gooey stuff), add the powder to the garlic footbath if desired.
3. Powdered marjoram: add to cornstarch and use as powder in socks, change socks 2-3 times a day and at bedtime.
4. Crush 3-6 garlic cloves, place in a jar, cover with olive oil, place in the sun or a warm place and steep for a week; apply to fungal areas three times a day.
5. Honey and garlic poultice to area 2-3 times a day.

6. Aloe Vera is soothing; apply after foot soak, air dry.
7. Vinegar to areas, do with sock changes.
8. This is what worked best for me when I had a ring worm infection on my hand. The infection was gone in just a few days: apply juice of lemon on the area 3-4 times a day. I also added a turmeric paste and covered the area with a band-aid.

BACK ACHE, MUSCLE ACHES, AND SPRAINS

Back ache and muscle aches:

1. Have on hand a bottle of sunflower or olive oil that has cayenne pepper or red chili powder in it; apply to area. It may hurt for a minute, but then gives relieve for 6-8 hours. Be sure and wash hands after applying.
2. Cloves (or clove oil): this will help relieve pain in the area. Make a strong tea with the clove buds, dip wash cloth into warm liquid and apply.
3. Parsley is a mild anti-spasmodic, make tea from the dried plant or juice the fresh plant, drink 3 times a day.
4. Apply ice or cold water compress for 15 minutes, then apply heat, alternate until pain and spasm relieved.
5. The Dineh (Navajo people) would heat a juniper branch, wrap it in deerskin or wool cloth, and place on sore area.
6. Celery seed teas calm and help relax, 1-2 cups a day.
7. Peppermint and thyme tea compresses, 2-3 times a day.
8. Try a relaxing hot bath with peppermint, thyme, or ginger, when my back was injured some years ago, I took a soak 2-3 times a day.
9. A compress of apple cider vinegar with salt added will help sore muscles, 2-3 times a day and add salt.

Ankle Sprain:

These are the most common injuries in America today. Without proper treatment you could face lifelong, chronic foot and ankle problems. A sprain occurs when you twist, turn, or roll your foot beyond its normal range. The ligaments are over stretched and may tear. Symptoms: bruising, tenderness, swelling, difficulty walking. **SEEK**

Jessie L. Emerson RN, Certified Clinical Herbalist

MEDICAL HELP if there is severe pain, numbness in foot or ankle, or the foot cannot move or bear weight, is pale or bluish color, feels cool to touch, if you hear a crunching sound on movement, there may be a fracture, any deformity of the joint may indicate a fracture. If a sprain doesn't improve in 72 hours of home treatment, Seek A Medical Practitioner. **CAUTION**: If you have osteoporosis, diabetes, nerve damage, or are taking blood thinners (baby aspirin is a strong blood thinner, don't be fooled by its name), seek professional help immediately.

Depending on the severity of the strain you will be at rest for 1-3 weeks. Your health-care practitioner will determine the best schedule for you. REMEMBER, the choice is up to you: adhering to the rest period recommended or cope with chronic pain, decrease in activity, and increase in money spent to control symptoms.

It is always better to prevent injury. See the index for exercises recommended by the American Academy of orthopedics.

Simple Sprains: You don't have to buy this R.I.C.E., just remember to use it:

1. **R**EST: take weight off the ankle.
2. **I**CE: do this immediately to keep swelling down. Wrap ice in towel or washcloth, if no ice, use cold water compress. Apply to area, leave on for 15 minutes, and do this 4 times a day. If you are diabetic or have nerve or blood vessel damage, use a cold-water compress and remove after 10 minutes.
3. **C**OMPRESSION: use an elastic wrap on ankle to support it and relieve swelling, but do not wrap too tightly and do not go to bed with it on.
4. **E**LEVATE: raise the foot to a level above your heart.
5. Anti-inflammatory: turmeric, basil, black pepper, cumin, and ginger—can be added to food, and eaten throughout the day. Ginger tea and green tea taste great and are stronger when used together. One can also take turmeric in capsules.

A compress of apple cider vinegar and salt will help sore muscles; do this 2-3 times a day, before or after an icing.
(For pain relief, see PAIN)
What is the most important therapy??? REST!

BLEEDING:

This may be the most distressing thing to observe but the simplest to control. First, where is the bleeding? Is the bleeding from an artery or a vein? An artery rapidly spurts bright red blood and requires immediate medical attention. **REMEMBER:** almost all external bleeding can be stopped with pressure, even an amputation or partial amputation.

1. Hold direct pressure by hand over a dressing. This prevents loss of blood while allowing normal blood circulation.
2. Hold the pressure for 15 to 20 minutes; if you think you have held long enough, hold for 5 minutes longer.
3. Do not peek under dressing, this disturbs blood clots and prolongs the blood flow.
4. If blood soaks through the pad, do not remove the pad; simply add additional thick layers of cloth or dressings.
5. Unless there is evidence of a fracture, the hand, neck, arm or leg can be elevated above the heart. This uses Earth's force of gravity to help reduce the loss of blood.
6. The pressure point method is used if direct pressure does not stop the bleeding. This technique stops circulation to the limbs and is held no longer than necessary to stop the bleeding. Continue the direct pressure and elevation. Reapply the use of the pressure point if bleeding recurs. Areas of the body where arteries pass close to the skin and over bones are called pressure points. Pressure applied at these points can inhibit or stop the flow of blood. Common pressure points:

   - Arm between the shoulder and elbow (Brachial artery).
   - Behind the knee (Popliteal artery).
   - Groin area (Femoral artery).

   To check if bleeding has stopped, slowly release your fingers from the pressure point. Be familiar with them before you have to use them.

7. The pressure dressing should not be so tight as to stop circulation. Observe frequently for blue fingertips and toes. If the victim is

conscious, ask frequently if they have numbness or tingling in toes or fingers.
8. Observe frequently for signs of continuous bleeding—blood soaking through and dripping.

Tourniquets are extremely dangerous and should only be applied when there is a life threatening hemorrhage, and should be applied only by a person experienced in the technique. REMEMBER, once it is applied you MUST seek care by a physician immediately.

BOILS AND CARBUNCLES:

Constant re-infection is a clue to reassess your lifestyle and diet. Something is affecting your immune system. Sores that do not heal and frequent infections can be signs of diabetes.

1. Wash area with vinegar and water.
2. White bread poultice; sprinkle a dash of cayenne or chili on bread, apply to boil 4-5 times a day; this usually opens and drains the boil.
3. After boil drains, wash with soap and water, apply antiseptic oils of: oregano, thyme, rosemary, or lavender to area with cotton ball and wear a dressing until drainage completely stops. Keeps clean, change dressing in the morning and before bed.
4. Do not forget to WASH YOUR HANDS.

BITES AND STINGS:

Prevention saves tears and time. Know and teach your children what harmful insects look like and where they like to live. Be respectful and avoid these areas when possible. Always be aware of your cohabitants on our planet Earth. Avoiding and repelling are better than killing. The sun shines on us all.

PREVENTION TIPS:

1. Store garbage away from house or campsite, keep lid on containers.

2. Do not approach garbage containers in bare feet or sandals.
3. Plant tansy to repel ants and other insects.
4. For removal of bee swarms, call a local bee keeper.
5. When camping, hiking, or attending outdoor activities, do not wear perfumes.
6. Light colored clothing attracts insects, especially bees.
7. Wear a hat; keep a net in your hat for encounters of the too close kind.
8. When outdoors, check beverage container before drinking (an absolute must).
9. When in tick country, inspect the body, scalp, and other hair covered areas daily; don't forget to inspect and brush dogs and pack animals.
10. Don't put your hands where you can't see, who knows what critter might live there.
11. Anyone known to have severe reactions to insect stings should carry epinephrine, in a kit or an "EPI" pen.
12. Wear herbal insect repellant before going outdoors.
13. Do not let a small child get into the face of a dog. Teach your child how to be around dogs. If a dog is acting strangely, drooling or is frenzied, avoid and report. There is a vaccine for rabies that no longer requires painful injections in the abdomen.
14. Be aware, prepared, and have FUN.

TREATMENT FOR BITES AND STINGS:

1. Do not use heat, this increases circulation and spreads the poison.
2. Apply ice but do not apply ice directly to skin. Wrap ice or ice pack in cloth and apply and reapply until swelling, redness, itching, or pain is relieved.
3. Prevent infection. Wash the area with soap and warm water or cider vinegar. Remove stinger from bee stings with tweezers.
4. Do not rub, scratch, squeeze or massage. This will increase swelling and spread the poison.
5. Apply a paste of baking soda and water to area to draw out the poison (if you have not green clay), leave on 15 minutes, brush off (do not wash off), and reapply if symptoms persist.

6. A poultice of white bread also works extremely well.
7. Wasps and mosquito bites can be treated by applying lemon juice, cider vinegar, lavender or cinnamon.
8. Apply poultice of crushed garlic or onion or both. In powdered form, garlic and cornstarch can be used as a bug repellant, especially for chiggers. Eating garlic daily also repels insects, but unfortunately it also repels some people.
9. Apply raw potato, turnip, or cabbage leaf as poultices, discard after 15 minutes, reapply if necessary.
10. Licorice powder will soothe the area.
11. Chamomile and mint tea will help nausea; sip until nausea is relieved.
12. Apply antiseptic spice oils sparingly: thyme, oregano, and lavender after washing and after poultices.
13. Treat symptoms as they arise.

BLADDER INFECTIONS:

What are you "pissed" about?
Treatment:

1. Water 8-10 8 oz. glasses per day.
2. Cranberry juice, pure, no sugar added, 6 oz. 3-4 times a day (can dilute with water).
3. Parsley tea, 2-3 times a day.
4. Corn silk: A tea of corn silk will soothe an inflamed bladder. When I prepare corn, I save and dry the silk, always having some in case there is a need, drink as often as needed.
5. Juice of: carrot, parsley, celery, cucumber, 2-3 cups a day.
6. Increase vitamin C intake, juice, or fruit.

BRONCHITIS:

This condition is an acute or chronic inflammation of the mucous lining of the bronchial tubes. Thick mucus may plug the swollen irritated bronchioles making if difficult to breathe.

Treatment:

1. Fenugreek tea several times a day.
2. Licorice tea: CAUTION. Do not use if taking steroids or blood pressure medicine, drink twice a day.
3. Thyme tea or thyme honey: Not for children under 1 year old. Expectorant, disinfectant, and soothes. To make, soak 1 oz. thyme in a pint of honey, leave in a warm place for two weeks, strain.
4. Onion tea: slice thin, cover with honey, steep at least 8 hours in covered container that you place in the sun, or in a warm spot in the kitchen Strain. Take a teaspoon every 3-4 hours. If you are totally isolated from people, or you don't really care who is around, you can add crushed garlic to the mix.
5. Old favorite: To warm water, add honey and lemon. Drink several times a day.
6. Anise tea: drink several times a day.
7. Steam inhalation of thyme or peppermint.
8. Drink the fresh juice of carrot, spinach, celery, beet, and/or cucumber daily.
9. Green tea daily.

BRUISES:

If you bruise easily, consult a health care professional. You could be vitamin deficient, experiencing side effects from anticoagulants, or have a medical condition.

Treatment:

1. Eat or juice dark green leafy vegetables.
2. Citrus and other fruits high in vitamin C and folic acid.
3. Potatoes, sliced thin and placed over bruise, 2-3 times a day.
4. Cabbage leaf over area, 2-3 times a day.
5. The traditional raw steak over the bruised and swollen eye. I really have never tried this, but people have told me it works.

Jessie L. Emerson RN, Certified Clinical Herbalist

BURNS:

Most burns can be prevented. Be Alert and Aware when around an open flame. Keep matches and lighters out of reach of children. Teach your children how to safely use matches or lighters. Turn handles of pans on stove toward the back of the stove, so children won't be tempted to reach for them. Don't use kerosene or other liquid flammables to light a fire, children watch and imitate—sometimes with serious results.

Burn basics:

1. Put the burned part into cold water or flush with cold water immediately, do not apply ice cubes.
2. Chemical burn: remove any chemical splashed clothing, flush or flood the area with cool water, do this for 30 minutes. Do not let rinse water get onto unaffected parts.
3. Leave blisters intact, they form a natural bandage, keeping bacteria out, body fluids in.
4. Keep as clean as possible to prevent infection.
5. Never put grease, animal fat, lard, coffee, mud, or feces on a burn. Remove any rings or shoes or constricted clothing; later there will be swelling that may make it difficult to remove them. If any clothing is stuck, don't try to pull off.
6. Give the severely burned person plenty of water; they can easily go into shock because of pain, fear, and loss of body fluids
7. Know the signs of shock (see shock).
8. If the person is conscious, give them the electrolyte drink, "Rehydration" 1 cup every hour if needed.
9. Treat the pain.
10. Treat inflammation.
11. See a medical person right away if the burn is more than a second-degree burn.

Types of burns:

1. First Degree: minor burns, outer layer of skin is bright red and painful—i.e. sunburn can usually be treated at home.

a. Cold water to affected area, or cold compresses, for ten minutes or until pain relieved.
   b. Spray or splash on apple cider vinegar and let evaporate every 2-4 hours as needed.
   c. Can use olive oil the next day to soothe.
   d. Aloe Vera: split open the leaf and apply the gel.
   e. Lavender oil: apply the next day.
   f. Fresh cucumber juice: if you can't juice, apply thin slices.
   g. Fresh live unsweetened yogurt will relieve the sting.
   h. Solution of sodium bicarbonate (baking soda); dip 4 x 4" gauze pads into solution and apply as often as necessary.

2. Second Degree: This type of burn makes a blister, keep intact. Same rules apply.
   a. Keep intact—everyone got that now? This is important.
   b. Olive oil, heat to boiling, cool to room temperature, test on inner wrist, place on dressing, and apply.
   c. Lavender or thyme oil: add to olive oil as bacteria static.
   d. Drink antibiotic teas: thyme, lavender, oregano, add honey.
   e. Aloe Vera gel: apply gauze dressing lightly, change daily. When my son was 3 years old, he burned the palm of his hand on a gas burner in the garage. I split a leaf of aloe vera, applied it to his palm and wrapped it in a dressing and applied an ace wrap. I changed this once daily. His palm healed, left no scarring, no contractures, and he was able to use his hand without any problems.
   f. Honey: cover area with honey; it soothes and prevents infection, especially staphylococcus; gently wash off and reapply twice a day.
   g. Tar burns: (Contributed by David RN) slather on mayonnaise, the mayo disintegrates the tar and makes it easier to remove (this is often used in the ER).

3. Third Degree: Destroys all layers of skin, is relatively painless (at first), may look white or charred. Follow all the burn basics.
   a. Cover large areas with gauze that has been dipped in solution of sterile water, salt, and bicarbonate of soda.
   b. If conscious, give fluids and Rehydration drink.
   c. A limb can be protected inside a clean plastic bag.
   d. Seek medical attention immediately.

COLDS AND FLU:

Viruses cause these. Antibiotics are given only for secondary bacterial infections. Stay home; don't infect others, especially babies, small children, and the elderly. Drink plenty of fluids. Wash your hands frequently. Sneezing, coughing into your hands, and then touching the eye can cause eye infections; cough into your elbow, the back of your hand, or into a tissue. A high fever, rapid shallow breathing, and pain in the chest when you breathe may indicate pneumonia. A visit to a health care professional is indicated. Prevention is the key. Garlic, onions, and cayenne included in the everyday diet can be your first line of defense.

1. Ginger tea: add lemon and honey or drink the following tea every 3-4 hours.
2. Grate fresh ginger root, 1 stick cinnamon, 1 tsp. coriander seeds, 3 cloves, 1 slice lemon, add to: 1-pint water.
3. Bring to a boil, simmer 15 minutes, strain, and sweeten with organic honey.
4. Make a strong ginger tea: dice ¼ of the fresh root, bring to a boil, then simmer 15 minutes. Add to a hot bath. Soak for 15-20 minutes, dry off, wrap in a wool blanket or sleeping bag, and "Sweat it out."
5. Onions: my mother always gave me little green onions to eat at the first signs of a cold. An old Missouri remedy is to steep a sliced raw onion in honey and eat throughout the day. You can also juice an onion and add the juice to the honey.
6. Citrus juice to increase Vitamin C in your diet.
7. Teas of: anise, fennel, parsley, peppermint.
8. Carrot juice (provides Vitamin A, the anti-infection vitamin).
9. Chicken soup: add 1-2 garlic bulbs, one onion, strain and drink the broth, can drink throughout the day.
10. Vegetarian soup: add garlic which is the main ingredient.
11. Licorice tea: helps the boost the immune system.
12. Snack on handfuls of pumpkin seeds throughout the day; contains zinc and will help the immune system.

CONSTIPATION:

Prevention:

1. Daily exercise: walking one hour a day works.
2. Water: 8 glasses a day.
3. Fiber: whole grains, salads, raw foods.
4. When the urge hits—GO.
5. Dottie's (my Mom) never fail remedy: warm prune juice in the morning just after awakening.
6. Warm water and lemon juice in the morning after awakening. Warm fluids and foods start the intestines moving.
7. Carrot, apple, celery, spinach, or grape juice—drink at room temperature daily.
8. This recipe is from *Back to Eden* by Jethro Kloss. Bran water daily: soak 1 cup bran in 1 quart water overnight;Strain and drink 1 cup in the morning.
9. Fenugreek seeds, flax seeds; 1-2 tsp. crushed and added to foods, very tasty in salads. If using this remedy, you must drink plenty of water to keep the bulk moving, more that 2 tsp. may cause abdominal distress, cramps, gas, or bloating.
10. Puree 3 stalks of rhubarb, add 1 cup apple juice, 1 tsp. lemon juice, honey to taste; this is powerful and should be used as last resort.

COUGHS:

Night coughs, night sweats, blood tinged sputum, are serious symptoms and require medical diagnosis. Proper coughing can prevent the spread of infection. Cover your mouth when you cough, teach your children these simple techniques. Turn your head away from people, cough into your shoulder, into the back of your hand or into a tissue or handkerchief. Coughing into your hand and then touching objects or people will spread infections. Wash your hands after coughing, sneezing, or blowing your nose.

1. Honey, lemon, and ginger tea, drink as needed.

2. Anise tea: 1-2 tsp. crushed seed added to boiling water, simmer 5 minutes and steep 15 minutes, add honey.
3. Thyme tea or thyme honey: soak fresh leaves in honey overnight, 1 oz. to 1 qt., strain and take throughout the day.
4. My mother used to rub my chest with "Vicks" (eucalyptus salve) and cover my chest with a piece of flannel; she also rubbed the bottom of my feet with the salve (she didn't know she was using reflexology).

CUTS, SCRAPES, AND ABRASIONS:

The main consideration is to prevent infection. A minor cut can turn into a major infection overnight. The skin is our largest organ; it keeps organisms out and us in. To stop bleeding, apply pressure for 5-10 minutes; when you think you have held long enough, hold one minute longer. Cleanse with soap and warm boiled water. Flood the area, or squirt the area gently with a bulb syringe or basting implement, washing out any foreign material. If the sides are wide open bring them together and bind with surgical tape. If it is a minor wound keep open. Above all, KEEP CLEAN.

1. Wash with a solution of vinegar and boiled water.
2. Apply honey and cinnamon.
3. Use one of these oils: clove, thyme, oregano, lavender, or rosemary.
4. I have dandelion in my kitchen garden; its leaves, crushed and mixed with water, make a soothing and drawing poultice.
5. Calendula, another kitchen garden plant, is used to reduce inflammation and promote wound healing.
6. Garlic: crush a clove and apply to area. If it irritates the skin, discontinue.

DIARRHEA:

Loose watery stools, gas, and cramping are the signs of diarrhea. I believe it is the body's attempt to eliminate poisons from the body. The main danger is dehydration, especially in infants, young children, and the elderly. Without treatment death can occur.

Causes of diarrhea:

1. Poor nutrition: poor nutrition causes diarrhea, diarrhea causes malnutrition; we must stop this circle—proper nutrition is important in preventing diarrhea.
2. Shortage of clean, uncontaminated water: unclean water contains the organisms that cause diarrhea and disease.
3. Intestinal flu.
4. Other infections in the body.
5. Malaria.
6. AIDS.
7. Inability to digest milk and other dairy products.
8. Allergies to certain foods (babies are often allergic to cow's milk and some artificial formulas, most baby foods contain GMOs).
9. Side effects from some medications.
10. Certain poisons: This may be from heavy metal contamination of the water or plutonium poisoning.
11. Laxative or purges gone awry.
12. Eating too much fruit, especially unripe fruit.
13. A baby is started on new food; mash the food well and mix with a little breast milk. Give in small amounts first. The baby's body has to learn how to digest new food. It is tough getting used to this planet. Go slowly.

DEHYDRATION:

Dehydration occurs when the body loses more liquid than it takes in. Many walk around in a semi-arid state every day. Our body was made to operate most efficiently in a water state, where electrolytes are in balance and at a certain temperature. When these conditions swing way out of balance, survival becomes an issue. It is lifesaving for everyone to know the signs of dehydration and how to treat it. However it is more important to prevent it from happening. When a person has watery diarrhea stool with or without vomiting, ACT QUICKLY. With children and elderly, there is no time to waste. Offer frequent sips of water. Keep them clean and dry to prevent loss of water through evaporation.

Signs of dehydration:

1. Thirst: in sub-clinical dehydration, thirst is often disguised by, "I am hungry." The next time you feel hungry; re-hydrate yourself with water or herbal tea. The herbal tea provides a boost in vitamins, minerals, and energy.
2. Little or no urine or the urine is dark yellow (this is also a sign of jaundice and hepatitis): without water our kidneys can't clean the waste products out of our body. Waste products accumulate and we become poisoned.
3. Sudden weight loss: our body is made up of 75-80% water; our bones are 25 % water.
4. Dry mouth: a chapped lip is just one of our body's cries for water, instead of a chapstick, drink water.
5. Sunken, tearless eyes: often people buy "tear drops" for their eyes, when maybe all they need is a glass of water.
6. Sagging in of the soft spot in infants: this is a dangerous sign, act quickly.
7. Loss of elasticity or stretchiness of the skin: gently take hold of the skin between two fingers; if when you let go, the skin does not fall immediately back to normal, the person is dehydrated.
8. Very severe signs: weak, rapid pulse, fast deep breathing, low blood pressure, fever, seizures, weakness, mental confusion, loss of consciousness.

When a person is weak from dehydration they may be too weak to care for themselves. Offer sips of liquids every 5 minutes until they begin to urinate and have light colored yellow urine. Offer the person frequent feedings of the foods listed. They may be too weak to take much at one time. Small frequent portions, along with frequent sips of liquid, are helpful and will produce positive results. It is also important to look at the cause of the diarrhea and treat the cause. Remember: if the diarrhea and/or dehydration become worse, seek medical attention because it may be necessary to give liquids and electrolytes directly into the vein, or medication may be required. However, most cases of diarrhea can be treated successfully at home—if you know what to do.

Treatment for dehydration

Rehydration: fluid replacement and electrolyte balance.
The Rehydration Formula:
    1 qt. boiled water that has been boiled for 10 minutes
    ½ tsp. table salt
    ½ tsp. baking soda
    1 tbs. fructose or you can add 3 tbl. honey or agave syrup to boiled water.

It is wise to keep container full of Rehydration mix, ready for instant use.

1. Drink 8-10 glasses of liquids a day, especially the "Rehydration Formula." A baby should nurse frequently. A good rule is an 8 oz. glass of water for every watery stool.
2. Eat ripe or cooked bananas, mash well, and add breast milk for babies.
3. Rice or oatmeal, if there is vomiting, rice or oatmeal water.
4. Apple sauce or well-cooked papayas.
5. Add cinnamon to applesauce.
6. Chicken or vegetable broth.
7. Mashed cooked carrots.
8. Cheese, if dairy is tolerated.
9. Yoghurt.
10. Teas: thyme, ginger, peppermint, chamomile; (peppermint and chamomile will also help painful cramping), epazote.
11. Honey in teas, except for children under 1 year of age.

DIZZINESS, MOTION SICKNESS:

Fresh air helps.

1. Ginger: drink ginger tea, carry candied ginger with you.
2. Celery seed: chew or make tea.

EARACHE:

When an infant or young child pulls at their ear, it usually means an earache. If you gently pull on the ear lobe, and there is increased pain, it is probably in the ear canal. If there is a sticky yellow-green discharge, there may be an acute infection of the middle ear. These are common and often can be prevented. Teach the child to wipe their nose, not to blow. If there is a stuffy nose, apply salt-water solution with a medicine dropper as needed. Breast-feeding is best. Do not let a baby fall asleep sucking on a bottle. The liquid goes into their ear. Never put a stick, wire, or similar object into the ear. My childhood doctor, Dr. MacDougal used to say, "Never put anything smaller than your elbow into your ear." Do not insert a cotton plug, let the infection drain out. If you think the eardrum has been perforated; if there is intense pain, partial loss of hearing, slight discharge of pus or blood lasting only a few hours, seek medical help. If acute pain persists longer than 48 hours, seek medical help. Hearing is more precious than gold or oil.

1. Clean out the ear using a bulb syringe, using warm water or peroxide, this will loosen any crusts and allow pus to drain.
2. Clean with warm boiled water and cider vinegar, 1 tsp. water, 1 tsp. vinegar, put vinegar and water drops in 4 times a day.
3. Apply garlic oil with a medicine dropper. Never put a clove directly into the ear.
4. Oregano oil: will help the pain and is an antiseptic.
5. Drink mint and chamomile tea.

EYE ISSUES:

Eye injuries should receive immediate attention. Even what one may think is a small injury can cause blindness if neglected. Foreign objects may be blown or rubbed into the eyes. Foreign objects that appear to penetrate the eye should only be removed or manipulated by an ophthalmologist (eye doctor).

Foreign objects—symptoms:

1. Burning sensation, scratching sensation, feels like something is in the eye.
2. Pain.
3. Photophobia (extreme sensitivity to light).
4. Tearing, over production of tears.

Precautions:

1. Keep from rubbing the eye.
2. Wash your hands before examining the eye, use gloves if available.
3. Copious irrigation; use 1 tsp. salt to 1 cup boiled and cooled water.
4. Removing object from surface of eye or inner surface of eyelid:
    a. Pull down the lower lid to see if the object is on the inner surface.
    b. If the object is on the inner surface, lift it gently with the corner of clean handkerchief or paper tissue. Never use dry cotton around the eye, moisten a cotton tip (use sterile water).
    c. If you cannot see the object, have the person look down; gently grasp the lashes of the upper lid.
    d. Pull the upper lid forward and down over the lower lid, tears may dislodge the object.
    e. Flush the eye.
    f. If the object cannot be removed, apply a dry protective dressing and consult a physician.

After the object is removed and the eye still feels scratchy, there may be a corneal abrasion. Cover the eye for 24 hours. NEVER cover an eye that has a discharge or pus. When the patch is removed, if the eye does not appear normal, seek medical attention.

Blunt Trauma to eye:

1. Examine eye after washing hands.
2. Treat with ice pack.

3. Keep person lying flat.
4. Cover with a dry sterile dressing or eye patch.
5. Seek medical help immediately.

Chemical Burns: *<u>This is a REAL emergency!</u>*

1. Immediate irrigation is essential for a minimum of fifteen minutes.
2. Identify the chemical, alkali is more serious than acid.
3. Seek medical attention immediately.

Pink Eye, Conjunctivitis:

This is an infection of the eye surface that is highly contagious. To prevent the spread among children, do not let a child with pink eye play or sleep with other children or use the same towel as other family members. It is usually self-limiting in two weeks.

Causes:

Bacteria: Generalized reddened look
Scratchy eyes
Discharge is pus
Matted shut after sleeping
Discomfort
Sensitive to light

Virus: Whites of eyes have blotchy red appearance
Discharge is watery, stringy
Discomfort
Sensitive to light

Allergic: Faint red or pinkish color
Discharge clear
Itchy eyes
May have runny nose and sinus infection

Treatment:

    a. Wash hands before and after working with the eye, use gloves if available. By now you know it would be proactive to have gloves with you in the home, in the car and in your backpack.
    b. Check eye to make sure foreign body isn't causing the symptoms.
    c. Irrigate the eye with fresh isotonic water 4 to 6 times a day using a fresh batch each time.

Isotonic solution is salt neutral, it matches our body, is neither too salty nor unsalty. Too much salt and the cells dehydrate and shrink; too little and they swell and burst.

To make isotonic solution:

    1 rounded teaspoon of salt for 1-quart water
    ½ teaspoon per pint
    ¼ teaspoon per 8-ounce cup
    Use sterile distilled water or boil first

Dip a cotton ball into the solution and drip the fluid into the eye.
Irrigate from inner eye to outer aspect to avoid reinvesting or contaminating with fresh bacteria.
Use a different cotton ball each time.
Do this 1 to 3 times at each irrigation.

    a. Compress: a warm compress of aloe vera juice is soothing and antibiotic.
    b. Antibiotic teas and spices: aloe vera, bay leaf, cinnamon, cloves, garlic, lavender (make into teas, or add to food).
    c. Anti-inflammatory spices: aloe vera, bay leaf, green tea, turmeric (make into teas or add to food).
    d. I believe one must go out of the kitchen for herbal remedies for pain and allergies.
    e. I would also suggest an antibiotic eye ointment (ophthalmic ointment).

f. If the eye doesn't improve or gets worse: increased pain, increase in swelling and redness, increase in pus or watery discharge, decrease in vision, see a health care practitioner immediately.

FAINTING:

Fainting is a partial or complete loss of consciousness due to a reduced supply of blood to the brain for a short time. To prevent loss of consciousness, any person who feels weak and dizzy should lie down or bend down with his head at the level of his knees.

Signs and Symptoms:

1. Extreme paleness
2. Sweating
3. Coldness of the skin
4. Dizziness
5. Numbness and tingling of the hands and feet
6. Nausea
7. Vision disturbances

What to do:

1. Ease the victim to the ground or if they have fallen, leave them there.
2. Turn them onto their side, turn head to the side.
3. Loosen constrictive clothing.
4. Bathe the face with a cool cloth.
5. Oil of peppermint under the nose.
6. Do not give any liquids if the person is unconscious.
7. Examine the victim carefully to see if they have suffered an injury from falling.
8. Unless recovery is prompt, seek medical assistance. Because fainting may be part of the development of a serious disease, the person should consult a medical professional.

FEVER:

Fever is a sign of illness. High fever is dangerous, especially in infants, small children, and the elderly. Do not give aspirin; salicylates in their isolated, concentrated from can cause a syndrome called Reyes Syndrome. Reyes syndrome can cause irreversible brain damage. If the fever is over 103, if it persists for over 2 days, seek medical assistance.

1. Do not bundle up a person with a fever. The less clothing the better. A tepid water bath, sponge bath, or wet cool towels applied to the neck and chest will lower the temperature.
2. Drink plenty of fluids, water, and herbal teas. If the urine becomes scant or concentrated, increase liquids.
3. Drink ginger tea. Pour a strong infusion into the bath of tepid water, use as cold compress, apply until fever breaks.
4. Peppermint tea.
5. Add cinnamon to teas.

FROSTBITE:

This is the result of frozen cells and tissues. The nose, cheeks, ears, fingers, and toes are most commonly affected. You can prevent this by using the "buddy" system. You and your buddy check each other's face often. If alone, cover your nose and exposed facial areas.

Signs and symptoms:

1. The area may become slightly flushed, later changing to white or grayish yellow
2. Loss of feeling in hands or feet
3. May have pain in the beginning but often it subsides
4. The victim may be unaware of his frostbite until he sees the pale, glossy skin
5. Tissue becomes hard as the cells freeze.

Treatment:

The object is to prevent further damage and to warm the affected area rapidly, maintain respirations and prevent refreezing. Seek medical attention as soon as possible.

1. Do not rub the injury with snow.
2. Do not rub the affected part at all, may cause gangrene (death of tissue).
3. Do not drink alcoholic beverages.
4. Do not smoke ANYTHING.
5. If you are not close to medical care, do not attempt to thaw a deep frostbite. If thawed and refrozen, this will cause more damage leading to amputations.
6. DO NOT apply heat lamp or hot water bottles.
7. DO cover the frozen part, provide extra blankets.
8. Give the victim a warm drink—a little cayenne in hot cocoa will get the circulation going, as will peppermint tea.
9. Immerse the effected part in warm water—between 102 and 105 degrees; take out of water immediately when area becomes flushed and gently pat dry. Place sterile gauze between the toes.
10. After the feet are thawed, do not let the victim walk on them. If the part is completely frozen, do not rewarm. Immobilize and get help immediately
11. Do have them wiggle fingers and toes to increase circulation.

GAS:

Undigested carbohydrates in the intestines produce most gas. Not being digested in the stomach, they sit in the small intestines until bacteria ferment them, thus producing "gas." Observe your diet; is it high in carbohydrates, artificial ingredients, or dairy products? Eliminate the offending foods. Slow down; chew your food more thoroughly. Gulping and using straws cause a person to swallow air. Lucky for us, the kitchen is full of spices and herbs that are gas relieving. Include them in your cooking or drink as a tea as needed.

1. Allspice, anise, basil, caraway, cardamom, cayenne, celery, cinnamon, dill, fennel, garlic, ginger, epizote, ginger, olive oil, oregano, papaya, parsley, peppermint, turmeric, thyme.

GOUT:

Redness, swelling, and pain in the extremities and joints, usually the big toe. Pain is worse on movement. This is caused by buildup of uric acids and it can cause severe pain. To reduce the chance of acute attacks: eat moderately, cut down on red meats and rich foods. Alcohol inhibits the excretion of uric acid. If fever is present, don't take aspirin; it also inhibits uric acid excretion. Include more fresh raw vegetables and fruit into your diet. If you suffer from chronic gout, consult your physician.

1. Increase water intake.
2. Chamomile tea.
3. Poultice of cayenne and oregano applied directly to joint, after initial "rush" will relieve pain 6-8 hours.
4. Turmeric—sprinkle on food daily, take capsules in acute stages.
5. Celery seed—eat celery on a regular basis.
6. Licorice tea.
7. Cherry juice—taken daily may prevent attacks.
8. Juice: carrot, celery, spinach, parsley, beet, cucumber.

HANGOVER:

I debated with myself whether or not to include this malady. However, it happens often enough to warrant inclusion. Too much alcohol causes dehydration, low blood sugar, irritation of the lining of the digestive track; it builds up acid in the blood, dilates blood vessels triggering headache and nerve pain plus mineral depletion.

Treatment:

1. Water, water, and water, at least 10 glasses if hangover is severe, add honey and lemon juice.

2. Juice: carrot, tomato, celery, onion, cayenne, garlic, black pepper; if only canned vegetable juice is available, add garlic, cayenne, black pepper and drink throughout the day—provides minerals and vitamins lost from alcohol metabolism.
3. Peppermint tea.
4. Black tea.
5. Onion soup—make with miso, add, guess what? Garlic, black pepper, cayenne; drink 1 to 2 cups or until symptoms relieved.

HEADACHE:

Everyone gets a headache now and again. About 90% are caused by tension. The other 10% are migraines, cluster, and caffeine withdrawal. If you suffer from migraines, note the foods you ate the day before and what chemicals you may have ingested or inhaled. (Read the labels: There may be chemical additives in foods that trigger migraines.) If headaches become chronic or severe, seek professional advice. For the occasional simple headaches try: relaxation techniques, deep breathing, and visualization.

Treatment:

1. Water, our best medicine.
2. Garlic, onions, and cayenne daily in your diet.
3. Ginger tea at onset of migraine, and then as needed.
4. Peppermint oil, lavender oil, thyme oil, rosemary oil applied to temples.
5. Relaxing hot bath at the onset, ginger tea can be added.
6. Thyme tea—hot compress applied to neck and shoulder muscles
7. Cinnamon, peppermint, and rosemary tea.
8. Bay leaf, basil, sage tea.
9. In New Mexico a bandana is soaked in cider vinegar and wrapped around the forehead. Often thin slices of white potatoes are soaked in vinegar and placed on the bandana and wrapped around the forehead.
10. This combination of juices has been found to help some migraines: carrot, spinach, celery, and parsley.

11. Caffeine—strong coffee or black tea taken at onset. This works most effectively if you do not drink large amounts of caffeine daily.

HEART ATTACK:

This is a life-threatening situation. Seek emergency medical treatment immediately. It is my belief that everyone should know CPR—it could save the life of a loved one.

Signs and symptoms:

1. Persistent chest pain, usually under the sternum (breastbone). The pain often radiates to one or both shoulders or arms, or elbow, or the neck or jaw or both. The pain may be very severe or mild; the degree of pain is not an indication of the seriousness of the disease.
2. Gasping or shortness of breath.
3. Indigestion, nausea, and vomiting; flu-like symptoms.
4. Extreme pallor or bluish discoloration of the lips, skin, and fingernail beds.
5. Extreme prostration.
6. Shock.

What to do:

1. Call 911; call for an ambulance.
2. Place in a comfortable position, usually sitting up, if extreme shortness of breath, use as many pillows as needed.
3. Loosen constrictive clothing.
4. If the victim is not breathing start CPR.
5. Never give liquids to an unconscious victim.

HEARTBURN/REFLUX:

Basic health rules apply here: eat slowly, chew thoroughly, remain sitting up after meals. Avoid excessive consumption of spicy foods, fried foods, processed foods, alcohol, and coffee. Do include more raw fruits and vegetables in your diet, especially those high in magnesium, such as fish (eat farmed fish—fish from the oceans are heavily contaminated with mercury and other poisons), apples, apricots, avocados, bananas, brown rice, garlic, kelp, lima beans, nuts, peaches, sesame seeds, green leafy vegetables, whole grains. Avoid negative conversation or thoughts during meals.

Treatment:

1. Water.
2. Apple cider vinegar, 1 tbl. mixed with water upon rising and/or with meals.
3. Aloe vera juice—one ounce, daily and as needed. It will soothe and heal the esophagus and mucus membranes of the digestive tract.
4. Sodium bicarbonate, short term use only.
5. Peppermint tea, chamomile tea, ginger tea, enjoy a cup after meals
6. Include these spices in your meals: cardomom, dill, fennel, caraway, marjoram, coriander.

HEAT EXHAUSTION/HEAT STROKE:

Always wear a hat when out in the sun. Infants, small children, the elderly, and those with no hair are especially vulnerable. We regulate heat and cold at the crown of our heads. Don't mow the lawn, run, or do any other physical activities at the hottest time of the day (12:00 noon to 4:00 pm). Wear a wet bandana around the neck to help keep the body temperature regulated at 98.6. <u>Heat exhaustion can quickly move to heat stroke</u>. Pour water over your head and the back of your neck. Drinking liquids can make the situation worse, cool down first.

Heat Exhaustion Symptoms: Weakness, dizziness, headache, profuse sweating, cool pale skin, rapid heart rate, mental confusion.

Heat Stroke: Sudden loss of consciousness, flushed, dry, hot skin, rapid irregular pulse, temperature may soar to 106-110 degrees.

1. Get victim out of the sun into a cool space.
2. Start chilling measures: tepid water sponge bath or ice bath, fanning, loosen, or remove clothing.

3. If conscious, give Rehydration Drink, ¼ cup every 15 minutes for 1 hour.
4. Medical care is urgently needed.

HIGH BLOOD PRESSURE:

A blood pressure greater than 140/80 puts a person at risk for heart attack and stroke. If it becomes chronic, kidney damage can occur resulting in the need for dialysis. Seek help from a health care professional to normalize your BP. Most high blood pressures can be controlled through a healthy diet and life style modifications, including stress management, counseling, anger management and daily exercise.

Signs:

1. Headache
2. Blurred vision, spots in the vision called floaters
3. Dizziness

In many cases, high blood pressure is silent, doing its damage undercover. This is why routine physical exams are important and recommended.

1. If extremely high, stay calm, lie quietly, and focus on your breathing.
2. Sip a tea made from 3 tsp. crushed celery seed. You can add chamomile, catnip, or skullcap herbs to the tea. A health care professional needs to be consulted at the earliest possible time.
3. If feet and legs are swollen, drink a cup of parsley tea, this will cause urination, taking the fluid load off the heart and therefore reduce the blood pressure.
4. Teas to help lower high blood pressure: Celery seed, chamomile, cardamom, fennel, and peppermint, green tea
5. A cup of "non salty" broth with ¼ to ½ tsp of the chili powder will help normalize blood pressure. Cayenne pepper increases force and strength of each heartbeat, dilates capillaries, and takes the load off the heart by increasing circulation to the hands and feet.

LOW BLOOD PRESSURE:

Evaluate. Is there adequate fluid intake? What medications are being taken? Is there a possibility of internal bleeding? Consult with your health care professional.

HYPOTHERMIA:

The lowering of body temperature faster than the body can produce heat. This often is caused by sudden emersion of the body into freezing water or being sprayed with cold water, or fuel and other liquids.

Symtoms:

1. Shivering may progress until the violent shakes are uncontrollable and the person is unable to take care of himself.
2. Core temperature falls to from 95 to 90 degrees; the person becomes sluggish, there is irrational reasoning, a false feeling of warmth may occur; if the temperature drops further the result is muscle rigidity, unconsciousness, and death.

The treatment:

1. Re-warm the whole body. Total body emersion should only be done in a hospital setting, because of the increased risk of cardiac arrest and re-warming shock.
2. Remove wet clothing.
3. Wrap in warmed blankets
4. Place in warm sleeping bag with another person who is already warm, skin to skin, no clothes. (The individual in the bag with the victim should not stay in the bag too long, or they could become hypothermic too.)
5. A warm sponge bath to the torso or place warm towels on torso and cover with blankets
6. If the victim is conscious, give them a warmed electrolyte drink with honey, or warm cocoa with added sweetener and cayenne.

7. When the victim is stable, seek medical assistance. There is the danger of re-warming too rapidly and then experiencing "after drop," the core temperature falls again to unsafe limits.

INFECTED WOUNDS:

The key here is PREVENTION. Wash the area, and keep clean. Inspect the wound twice a day. Signs of infection: redness, swollen, hot, painful, fever, redline or streaks going away from the wound, swollen under lymph nodes, bad smell, pus.

Signs of Gangrene:

Very bad smell, like dead flesh, brown or grey liquid oozes out, skin turns black, air bubbles or blisters. Seek medical attention immediately

For puncture wounds, wash thoroughly, apply white bread poultice, and seek medical attention immediately. For large wounds, abdominal wounds, gunshot wounds, animal or human bites, you guessed it— ***SEEK MEDICAL ATTENTION IMMEDIATELY.***

Treatment to Prevent Infected Wounds:

1. Warm or hot, wet compresses over wound 4 times a day.
2. Compresses may be made with: cinnamon and honey, apple cider vinegar, oregano, chamomile, peppermint, lavender.
3. Drawing poultices: white bread, cabbage leaves.
4. After compresses: apply aloe vera, oil of oregano, clove, lavender, or thyme.
5. Increase Vitamin C in your diet to enhance your immune system.

INSOMNIA:

When this becomes a chronic problem it would be wise to see a health care professional to learn and treat the underlying cause.

1. Have you been getting enough fresh air and exercise during the day? Go outside take 10 deep slow breaths and count your blessings. Do some relaxing yoga.
2. Take a relaxing hot bath.
3. These teas will help: chamomile, celery seed, cilantro, basil, thyme.
4. If you can't sleep: clean those kitchen cupboards you've been putting off doing, read a scientific book on how nanotechnology works.
5. Keep an herbal remedy around, like catnip, pasaflora, or valerian; for just such occasions, something stronger than celery seed may be needed.
6. Set the alarm and wake up same time every day, regardless of when you fell asleep—finally dropped off at 4:30 AM—wake up at usual time.
7. Have a physical check up, there may be a physical cause.

MORNING SICKNESS

1. Ginger tea, ginger candy, throughout the day as needed.
2. Soda crackers—sometimes helps if eaten when you first wake up.
3. 1 tsp. bee pollen in fruit juice daily; B complex vitamins will help, but a pill may be too strong—bee pollen is more gentle and also contains other nutrients.
4. Spearmint tea—peppermint tea may be too strong and could cause miscarriage in some women.
5. Eat a snack an hour before you go to bed.

NOSEBLEEDS:

If a nosebleed occurs after a blow to the head, it may be a sign of a skull fracture. Stay calm, sit quietly, and seek medical help.

1. Grasp the soft part of the nose firmly and hold firmly for 10 minutes, then for another 2 minutes. Don't blow the nose, may dislodge the clot and start the bleeding again.
2. Cold compress to back of neck.

3. Apply witch hazel to piece of cotton, insert inside the nose leaving a tail, keep in for at least an hour. Doesn't everyone keep witch-hazel in the kitchen? If not, it might be a good idea.

PAIN:

There are two kinds of pain: acute and chronic. Chronic pain persists for weeks and months. Do not ignore pain; it is the body getting your attention, trying to communicate, "Something is wrong." Find out what it is.

1. Turmeric for arthritis pain—take 1 to 2 capsules several times a day or sprinkle daily on food.
2. Rosemary tea.
3. Peppermint or lavender oil externally, place on the temples for headaches
4. Hot pack alternating with cold packs for 15 minutes to painful aches and sprains, apply as often as needed.
5. Cayenne poultice to area; it blocks the pain signals that come from the nerves just under the skin. It also prevents nerve cells from making more pain signal cells.
6. Drink a cup of dill, chamomile, or lavender tea when the cramps of colic begin.

POISON IVY, OAK, OR SUMAC:

Learn to recognize and avoid. However, I did have an uncle who became ill from inhaling the volatile oils of one of these plants when a patch was burned by a neighbor. Don't scratch, it will spread or cause an infection. If lung is involved, seek medical help.

1. Wash area with mild soap and water, taking care not to let it drip on unaffected parts of body.
2. Bathe area with cider vinegar.
3. Squeeze the juice of aloe vera leaf on area.
4. Paste of oatmeal made with cool water and applied; it will soothe. Paste of sodium bicarbonate; gently wash and reapply throughout the day.

5. Green tea: internal and as a compress helps inflammation.

SHOCK:

Shock is life threatening. There are many causes: large burns, major blood loss, dehydration, severe allergic reactions, and heavy bleeding inside the body.

Signs of shock: weak rapid pulse, cold sweat, pale, cold, clammy skin, blood pressure low, weakness, mental confusion. At the first sign of shock or if the person is at risk of shock:

1. Have the person lie down, the feet a little higher than the head.
2. Cover with a blanket.
3. Stop any bleeding.
4. If conscious, give the electrolyte Rehydration Drink.
5. Seek medical help immediately.

SEIZURES:

A seizure or convulsion is usually attributed to a neurological malfunctioning, sometimes violent in nature. However, there are milder forms that may only be brief momentary loss of contact with the surroundings. They can occur with someone who has epilepsy or be the result of infection, high fever, or be associated with head injury or brain or nervous system disorders.

Signs and symptoms:

1. Rigidity of body muscles, usually lasting from a few seconds to perhaps a minute; this is followed by jerking movements.
2. The victim may stop breathing.
3. Bluish discoloration of the face and lips.
4. May bite tongue.
5. Foaming at the mouth or drooling.
6. Loss of bladder and bowel control.

Treatment:

1. Prevent the victim from hurting himself.
2. Do not restrain or hold down.
3. Do not place a blunt object into the mouth.
4. Do not pour liquids into the mouth.
5. Do not place a child in a tub of water.
6. Give artificial respiration if indicated.
7. When the seizure has subsided, place the person on their side, turn head to one side, to allow secretions to drain and prevent choking.
8. Cover and keep warm. The person may be weak, slightly confused, or want to sleep
9. Call for medical help if seizures persist without stopping, any injuries occur, or of the person continues in a state of confusion.

SINUSITIS:

This infection and inflammation may come after a cold or allergy attack or be associated with a dental infection. If it persists or becomes chronic, seek medical help.

1. To one cup boiling water, add 7 drops peppermint oil, and inhale the steam. This remedy is from the Native American herbalist Rolling Thunder. Don't drink this—never take internally the "oils" of any herbal product.
2. Peppermint or oregano tea, inhale, may drink.
3. Nose drops or salt and water; use medicine dropper, or wet a cotton ball and squeeze into nose or use a netti pot.
4. A taste of horseradish or hot salsa made with cayenne will usually open the sinuses.
5. Be sure to include garlic and cayenne in your meals.

SPLINTERS AND SLIVERS:

Do not ignore as they can become infected. If you have diabetes, do not attempt self-remedy, see your primary care doctor.

1. Wash the area with mild soap and water; if water source is questionable, boil the water and let it cool.
2. Try to pull out with tweezers.
3. If just under the skin, sterilize a needle by heating the point in a clear point of a flame for several minutes, allow to cool and EASE the splinter out.
4. Do not dig deep with unsterile implements.
5. I keep a jar of pine sap in my cupboard, soften it and place over area, hold on with Band-Aid, it will draw it out (from personal experience).
6. A white-bread poultice.
7. If the splinter is glass or embedded deeply, a medical person should be seen.

SORE THROAT:

1. Gargle with warm water, salt, and cayenne.
2. Honey and lemon drink.
3. Drink your antibiotic teas, every 4 hours for the first few days, and then you can taper to every 8 hours; add honey and a dash of cinnamon.

STROKE:

A stroke usually involves a clot in a blood vessel to the brain or a rupture of a blood vessel in the brain. Prompt medical attention is necessary. This is an emergency situation and time is of the essence.

Signs and symptoms:

1. Paralysis or weakness on one side of the body.
2. Difficulty breathing and swallowing.
3. Slurring of speech or unable to talk.
4. One side of the mouth droops; ask person to smile if you think they may have had a stroke—if one side of the mouth droops that is an indication.
5. Pupils unequal in size.
6. Loss of bladder and bowel control.

7. Headache.
8. Confusion.
9. Slight dizziness and ringing in the ears.
10. Memory changes.
11. Disturbance in the normal personality.
12. Unconsciousness.

Treatment:

1. Protect the patient from accident; position on side, head to one side.
2. Cover with blanket.
3. Loosen clothing.
4. Maintain open airway.
5. Begin CPR if there is no pulse.
6. Do not give fluids even if the person is conscious, the throat muscles may be paralyzed, allowing the liquid to go into the lungs.
7. Call for medical help immediately.

TOOTHACHE:

Why does it always happen in the middle of the night?

Treatment:

1. Cloves:
   A. Chew on a few pieces of dried cloves, place next to painful tooth.
   B. Make a strong tea of cloves, dip a small piece of cotton into the tea and place on the tooth where the pain is.
2. Then make that appointment to see the dentist that you have been putting off for a while.

TIPS ON HOW TO DO IT

I have included some basics, such as how to boil water, as some who read this book may be novices in the kitchen—we all have to start sometime and somewhere. But do not wait for an emergency. Become familiar with these before the need arises so you will be calm and competent.

BOIL WATER:

Drinking water must be protected from contamination, especially from the feces of animals and humans. Contaminated water is often the cause of diarrhea, which can be fatal in babies and the elderly. It is best to keep a supply of purified water on hand to use in emergencies or disaster situations. If you suspect your water has become contaminated, do not even use it to brush your teeth. Boiling water kills bacteria, viruses, and parasites. Boiling water is the more effective water purification method than treating it with chlorine bleach or other chemicals. The best type of containers to store water is glass containers that have tight fitting screw caps. The containers should be disinfected before filling them with purified water. You can either do this by using bleach or pour boiling water into the container. Do not boil plastic containers. To use bleach: pour 1 tablespoon of liquid bleach to one gallon of water; pour into the container to be disinfected; let it set for 10 minutes; pour out the solution; rinse with purified water; and pour out the rinse water. Pour in the purified water, cap. The water must be used within 6 months.

To boil containers for disinfecting: in a large pan, submerge the glass container; bring to a rolling boil and then boil for 10 minutes.

Boiled water:

Water boils at 212 degrees at sea level. The higher the altitude, the lower the atmospheric pressure. The less atmospheric pressure, the easier it is for water molecules to escape into the air. Water comes to a boil quicker at higher altitudes. The boiling point of water is higher on a stormy day and will take longer to come to a boil. Choose a pot that's large enough to hold the water you want to boil. A short wide pan will come to boiling point sooner than a tall narrow one.

1. Use cold water.
2. Do not fill the pot all the way up, boiling water increases in volume.
3. Put on stove or campfire or hot coals.
4. Placing a lid on pan speeds the process.
5. When you see steam coming out of the lid, water is soon to boil.
6. Bubbles indicate water is boiling; wait for the bubbles that rise to the top of the pot.
7. Slow boil: 205 degrees, noticeable movement with large bubbles.
8. Rolling boil: 212 degrees, the water is rolling, vigorously bubbling and steaming.

If you are purifying water it must boil for 10 minutes, make sure there is enough water in the pan.

COMPRESSES:

External application that is usually dipped into an herbal solution, or vinegar, that is used to treat superficial ailments, stimulate circulation of blood or lymph, relieve colic and muscle spasms, reduce inflammation, reduce fevers, and restore vitality. Two rules to remember: 1. If the affected area is red and hot, apply warm moist compresses. 2. If the affected area itches and oozes clear fluid, use cold wet compresses.

1. Boil water and allow it to cool until you can just put your hand safely into it, 100 to 108 degrees.
2. Make an herbal tea, use plain water or vinegar.
3. Dip a towel or cloth into the water or strained tea.
4. Squeeze out the extra liquid.
5. Apply as hot as can be tolerated, but no more that 115 degrees.
6. Cover with a dry flannel cloth.
7. When it begins to cool, apply another warm compress and repeat the process.

COUGH SYRUP:

Syrup is used for coughs, throat inflammations, and to soothe the stomach and intestinal tract. Syrup can be made with honey or sugar. Natural, local, unprocessed, and unheated honey is the best choice. CAUTION: Honey is not given to infants or children under 1 year of age. I have included both honey and sugar recipes. It is a wise idea to make these up in advance, and be prepared.

Preparation of honey syrup:

1. Two ounces of herbs
2. One quart water
3. Boil gently, reducing to 1 pint
4. Strain
5. While still warm (below 98.5°F) add 2 to 4 ounces of honey

Making a stronger syrup:

1. One gallon honey
2. Four cups total herbs and tie in a cheesecloth
3. Bring to boil
4. Turn down to a simmer for one hour, maybe thinned with purified water if too thick

Simple Syrup, using sugar, makes 1 quart:

1. Place 14 ounces sugar into blender
2. Add 14 ounces of water and blend on high for about 3 to 4 minutes
3. Add another 8 ounces of herbal tea and blend another 1 to 2 minutes
4. Add another 14 ounces of sugar and blend
5. Simple syrup is safe for children under 1 year.

HERBAL BATHS:

There are baths for every purpose and several ways to prepare your bath.

1. Place a handful or about ½ cup of herbs in cheesecloth or washcloth and tie; place in cotton muslin bag or large rice cooking ball and place in the tub under the running water. Lacking any of these items you can just add the herbs to the bath being careful not to clog up the drain.
2. Place the herbs in a covered nonmetal pot, cover with water. Bring to a boil and simmer covered for 10-20 minutes. Strain the material and pour the liquid into your tub.
Soak for at least 20 minutes. Enjoy, relax, and do not forget to compost the plant material.

MUSTARD PLASTER:

This is a well-known folk remedy that has been used for hundreds of years. Placed on the chest, it breaks up congestion, relieves asthma, bronchial pneumonia, and pleurisy, and eliminates coughs, head colds and flu. It can be used to treat sprains and painful joints. Mustard seeds, Sinapis alba, are rubefacients, bringing circulation to the skin and thereby bringing heat, nutrition, and oxygen. CAUTION: The actual paste NEVER comes into direct contact with the skin. If left on too long, it can blister the skin so do not put on sensitive places. Mustard plasters should not be used on children under 6 years.

1. Mix 4 tbl. flour and 1 tbl. of powdered mustard seed (if using wild mustard seed, use 2 tbl. seeds). Now is the time to use your mortar and pestle.
2. Mix with enough cold water to make a thick paste.
3. Spread paste on cotton, flannel, or hemp cloth.
4. Place a thin cloth on the skin.
5. Place mustard cloth on top of the thin cloth.
6. Leave on 10 to 15 minutes or until skin begins to redden and has a tingling sensation.
7. Encourage patient to drink plenty of liquids.
8. A warm or cool shower afterwards promotes rest.

POULTICE:

A warm moist mass of powdered herbs that is applied directly to the skin to:

1. Relieve inflammation
2. Draw out poison from venomous bites and stings
3. Skin eruptions
4. Promote proper cleansing and healing of affected area

Fresh or dried herbs can be used.

1. Grind the herbs to a powder. For fresh herbs, simmer two ounces in half a pint of water for 2 to 3 minutes; pour the entire mixture into a cheesecloth.
2. Moisten the powdered herbs with hot water.
3. Gently wash the area with soap and water.
4. Place a thin cloth over area.
5. Apply the herb mixture, may also be applied directly to the skin.
6. Cover with another cloth or towel to retain the heat.
7. Apply a fresh poultice when it cools.
8. Gently wash the area after removing the poultice.

STEAM INHALATION:

Inhalation consists of warm moist air brought to the mucous membranes of the respiratory tract. This treatment:

1. Relieves inflammation and congestion of the mucous membranes of the upper respiratory tract.
2. Relieves dry throat tickle by moistening the air.
3. Loosens secretions and stimulates expectoration.
4. Relaxes muscles, relieves coughing.
5. Prevents excessive drynes of mucous membranes.
6. Relieves stress headaches.
7. Relieves clogged sinuses.
8. Relaxes the mind and calms the spirit.

CAUTION:

1. Pay attention. The water needs to boil and can scald if proper precautions are not taken.
2. Keep children and pets away while taking the treatment.
3. Be especially careful when giving treatment to children or restless patients.

Equipment:

1. Filtered or purified water
2. Kettle or pot
3. Glass or ceramic bowl or tall tea pot
4. Herbs or essential oils
5. Towel
6. To make a croup tent, open an umbrella, place sheet over umbrella to form a tent.

Directions:

1. Heat water until it steams.
2. Pour over herbs in container or pour water and add essential oils.
3. Place towel over head so it forms a tent.
4. Lean toward the steam, being careful not to get too close.
5. Inhale slowly and deeply.
6. Treatment lasts 15 to 30 minutes.
7. If you or the patient starts to feel overheated or uncomfortable, remove the towel or sheet.

TEA:

Read Tea Tips.
Now you are ready to make your tea.
Use leaves and flowers (an infusion):

1 tsp. of dried leaves or 20 fresh leaves or flowers.
To steep, pour boiling water over herbs, cover and steep for 3 to 5 minutes.
Roots, bark, or seeds (a decoction):
1 tsp herb, 2 cups boiling water, simmer 5 to 10 minutes; to make stronger, leave covered for 6 hours or overnight.

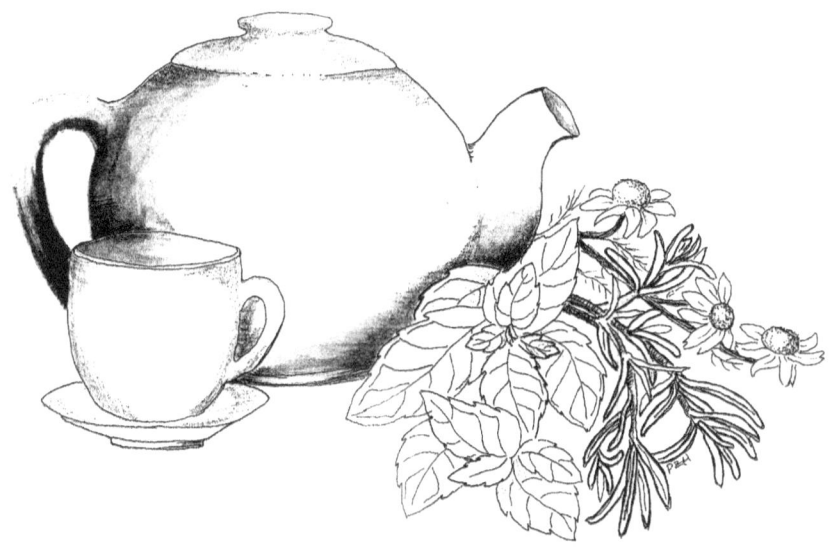

MY FAVORITE TEAS TO KEEP IN THE KITCHEN

These are my favorite teas that have helped me through many unexpected circumstances. I have also included one juice that now goes with me everywhere.

1. **TEA:** *Camellia sinensis*, black and green. Confused about these teas? All teas, both black and green, come from the same plant Camellia sinensis. The difference in the teas is the way the leaves are processed. Green tea is the least processed. Black tea is fully fermented; the leaves are exposed to air causing oxidation. This makes the leaves a rich brown color. Both are sources of Vitamin C: one cup equals 3 glasses of orange juice. Green tea is rich in fluoride and is antimicrobial, a combo that both prevents and heals gum disease. (Research has shown that

gum disease can cause heart disease, stroke, and diabetes.) Both green and black teas contain tannins and flavinoids, which is why they are helpful in skin conditions. A tried and true remedy for nursing mothers is placing a wet and cool tea bag on sore breasts and nipples. Tea is an age-old home treatment for burns, wounds, and sunburns. A poultice relieves itching and inflammation from insect bites. A compress stops bleeding. My grandmother Grace used to make me a cup of tea when I had an upset stomach. Milk does not adversely affect the absorption of the constituents of tea—so add your cream and sweetener and enjoy.

2. **CATNIP:** *Nepeta cataria*, leaves. Every cat owner has at least one catnip mouse, complete with fake whiskers, lying around the house. No, I am not suggesting you raid your pet's toy. Fresh catnip from your garden is best. Although it excites cats of all ages, it is an effective muscle relaxant for us humans. Can't sleep? Mind still jogging after the day at work? Add some skullcap to the catmint, and sip on your tea while you take a nice hot lavender bath. Catnip is somewhat bitter; I add honey, stevia, or agave syrup to sweeten the taste.

3. **CHAMOMILE:** *Matricaria recutita*, flowers. When you need an herb to calm down, chamomile is the number one choice. It is effective for anxiety, palpitations, and all manifestations of stress, including insomnia. Because it has no side effects or toxicity, it is safe for babies who are suffering from colic. (Remember no honey until the child is a year old.) People who are allergic to pollen may not be able to take chamomile. At first sign of cold or flu drink Chamomile tea; it is antibacterial, especially against staph aureus and streptococcus. It is also lowers a fever.

4. **CHAPARRAL:** *Larrea tridentate*. Okay. I admit not too many people keep Chaparral tea in their kitchen, and even less actually drink it. I am never without it. Fighting an infection, drink chaparral. Do you have joint pain, arthritis? Start drinking a cup a day and notice your improvement. I find it especially useful

for bronchitis and coughs. When young, my granddaughters would sleep with a glass of chaparral by their bedside. They would wake up coughing, take a drink, and then sleep until morning.

5. **GINGER:** *Zingiber officinale.* Drink a cup when you have a queasy stomach or indigestion. Make a stronger cup at the first sign of cold, flu, or fever to prevent the condition from going deeper into your body. Make a strong tea of grated fresh ginger, i.e.—steep for 15 to 20 minutes, add it to a tub of hot water and take a long soak. After your bath, wrap yourself in blankets to further "sweat out" the fever. (From Brenda Morales Montoya, RN and DOM).

6. **LAVENDER:** *Lavandula officinalis.* If I had limited space, I would definitely always have lavender and mint. Even smelling lavender energizes and lifts spirits. Stuffed up with a head cold or allergy? Inhale lavender steam. Lavender is a plant of many uses: soothes nerves, is antispasmodic and therefore useful for gas and dyspepsia, heartburn, or reflux. It is safe for infants under 6 months (I like chamomile for older children). I also keep lavender oil to use as "smelling salts." When the going gets tough, the tough sip lavender tea.

7. **MINT:** *Mentha piperita*, all mints. I am never ever without mint. My favorite is Poleo, Mentha arvensis, or high mountain mint. When I drink it, I am immediately transported to a high mountain stream and I immediately relax and "cool it." The uses of this plant are many: antispasmodic, carminative, upset stomach, anti-inflammatory, anti-bacterial, inhale for excessive mucus in respiratory systems, it calms and quiets; in aroma therapy, it is used to increase concentration.

8. **ROSEMARY:** *Rosemarinus officinalis.* Cannot remember what you need when you are at the grocery store? Make a list. Cannot remember where you put the list, or the car keys? Time for a cup of Rosemary Tea. Rosemary aids the memory and helps keep the mind alert—without the nervous energy and unfocused

actions of caffeine. It is an excellent remedy for headaches, nervousness, and nervous indigestion. No get up and go in the mornings? Forget the caffeine rush. A nice energizing rosemary bath followed by a cup of rosemary tea will energize and focus you for the day's activities. It has been used to increase poor circulation and strengthen fragile blood vessels. Oh, and don't forget its use as a hair tonic.

9. **ROSEHIP:** *Rosa spp.* Nothing is more beautiful than the wild rose. It can be found in all altitudes, but most frequently in mountainous areas, streamside, and moist meadows. The flowers mature into hips, the little fruits that turn from greenish yellow to a translucent dark red. Rosehips are a local and inexpensive source of Vitamin C. They have 60 times the Vitamin C as citrus fruit. They are also a source of bioflavonoids that aid in the absorption of Vitamin C and iron. The seeds can be ground into meal and added to cereals and muffins. They are a source of vitamin E, sulphur, and unsaturated fats. Add a little cinnamon and enjoy on a cold winter day.

10. **ALOE VERA:** *Aloe barbadensis.* Technically, this is not a tea. However, I drink its juice daily and always have a plant available for burns. The gel heals cuts and burns and the juice soothes and heals an irritated digestive tract. It is anti-bacterial and anti-inflammatory.
This plant has many nutritional compounds in abundance and it is high in magnesium (magnesium is the main compound in many of the over-the-counter reflux and heartburn pharmaceuticals).
I prefer to prevent or heal disease using natural remedies because there are fewer side effects, and I save money.

TEA TIPS

Loose teas are preferred, as some of the delicate and subtle flavors can be lost in bags. Herbs you pick yourself or that are picked by someone you know insures that they have been gathered in a positive and thankful way, have not been irradiated and have not been contaminated with pesticides and herbicides. Fresh herb tea from your garden is a special treat.

Teas should be stored in airtight containers in a cool dark place. Fresh herbs are chopped or used whole. Use one tablespoon or 20 to 25 leaves. Crush seeds before brewing to bring out flavor. Roots are crushed or chopped. Avoid using stems for most plants, i.e.—mint, stems add a stronger more bitter taste; however when using the southwest plant, Cota (*Thelesperma spp*), flowers, leaves, and upper stems are used. Know Your Plant. Fresh or dried herbs can be added to black teas for additional flavor. Use pure water or filtered water. Note the difference when spring water is used. Herbal teas and sun tea go together.

- Boil water until it is bubbling and rolling frantically. Rinse teapot or cup with hot water, add the tea and cover with the boiling water. Cover the tea while it steeps; this will prevent the aroma and medicinal properties from being carried away in the steam.
- Steep 3 to 5 minutes. Steeping longer may release bitter flavors from chemical constituents in the plants, i.e.—tannins, alkaloids.
- When trying a new tea or herb, test for sensitivity by taking a small quantity first. If it makes you sick, take less or throw it away. When taking plants for therapeutic reasons, if it doesn't work, take more, if it still doesn't work, stop taking it. Too much can also hurt. Do as directed. Do in moderation. If you don't get better, or if you get worse, call your health care professional. Above all, Trust Your Own Judgment.

Sweeteners can be used such as honey, raw sugar, maple syrup, molasses, stevia, or agave syrup. Milk distorts the flavor. Try first without any additions to taste the real flavor. Try lemon, lime, or orange slices. Artificial sweeteners, such as aspartame are poison to the body and should be avoided.

Make your own personal teas: a tea for a rainy day, for those 100 degree days, to perk you up after a hard day at work, girl-talk teas, a special tea for that special someone in your life, to enhance those natural desires, a relaxing tea. For every occasion there is a tea.

Grow your own teas for your special blends. Outdoor garden or window garden, they will brighten your life and become your friend. Seeds from native plants can be gathered or obtained from various seed companies or organizations specializing in wild plants.

Above all, have fun and stay healthy.

LIST OF SPICES—MEDICINAL USES

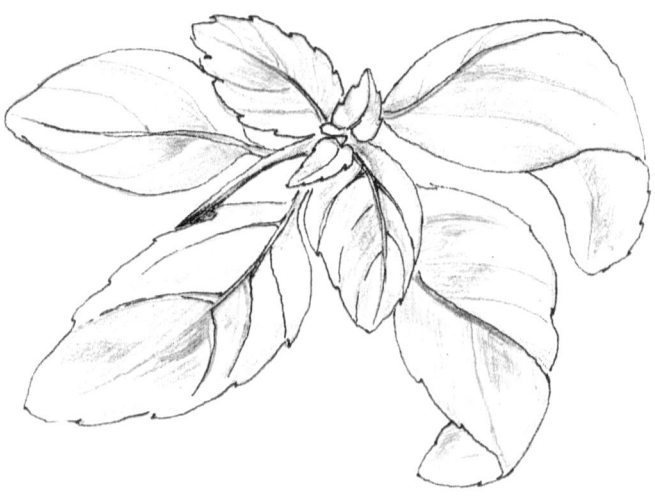

ANISE: *Pimpinella anisum*
    Part used: seeds
    Use: Aids digestion, colic, gas, carminative, coughs, promotes expectoration, bronchitis, spasmodic asthma, the oil is used as antiseptic, repels insects.

BASIL: *Ocimum basilicum*
    Part used: leaves
    Use: Carminative, mild nervous disorders, fresh leaves placed on stings draw out poison, insect repellant, mild antiseptic.

BAY: *Laurus nobilis*
    Part used: leaves, oil
    Use: Aids digestion, colic, diuretic, arthritis, inflammations, antioxidant, protects cardio-vascular system, bacterial and fungal infections, high blood sugar, inhibits growth of cancer cells.

CARDAMOM: *Elettaria cardamomum*
    Part used: dried ripe seeds
    Use: digestive system: carminative, dyspepsia, indigestion, helps stop belching, vomiting; respiratory system: added to milk to neutralize the mucus forming properties, expectorant; calms nervous system; detoxes caffeine, calms nervous stomach.

CAYENNE: *Capsicum annum*
    Part used: whole fruit
    Use: anti-viral, increases circulation, brings blood from center of body to periphery, helpful in congestive heart failure; blood to mucosa, counter irritant, diaphoretic, stimulates production of hydrochloric acid, salivary and intestinal juices, doesn't irritate lower digestive tract; reduced uric acid, diuretic, relieves pain.

CELERY: *Apium graveollens*
    Part used: seed, leaves, and root
    Use: carminative, diuretic, stomach tonic, calms nerves, good for hysteria, promotes sleep.

CHIVES: *Allim schoenaprasim*
    Part used: leaves
    Use: stimulates appetite, digestive aid, high in iron and sulfur, calcium, magnesium, potassium, thiamine and niacin, mildly antibiotic, high concentrations of vitamins A and C, tones stomach, reduces blood pressure.

CHOCOLATE: *Theobroma cacao*
    Part used: bean, bark, made into butter fat
    Use: mild stimulant to nervous system, asthma, bronchitis, respiratory distress, anemia, antioxidant, mood calming; and for those intimate moments, increases virility.

CILANTRO: *Coriandrum sativum*
    Part used: fruit and leaves
    Use: stimulant aromatic, carminative, anesthetizes stomach, digestive aid, soothing laxative, soothes cramping, seeds as sedative.

CINNAMON: *Cinnamonum zeylanicum*
    Part used: dried bark
    Use: high in calcium, menstrual cramps, digestive aid, flatulence, diabetes, astringent, diarrhea, antibacterial, inhibits e-coli, staph aureus and candida albicans.

CITRUS: *Citirius aurantium, Citrus vulgaris* (lemon, lime, orange, etc)
    Part used: fruit, peel, and flowers
    Use: anxiety and nervous depression; stimulates digestive juices, diuretic, fruit high in Vitamin C, antioxidant.

CLOVES: *Eugenia aromatic*
    Part used: underdeveloped flowers
    Use: anesthetic, germicide, antiseptic, antithelmic.

COFFEE: *Coffea arabica*
    Part used: berries, seeds, leaves
    Use: stimulates the central nervous system, has a "wake up" effect on the brain, diuretic.

CORN SILK: *Zea mays*, maize
    Part used: silk
    Use: diuretic, acute and chronic cystitis, irritation of uric acid and phosphate gravel, emollient poultice for ulcers, swelling, rheumatic pains, nausea, and vomiting.

CUMIN: *Cuminum cynimum*
    Part used: seeds
    Use: curry and spice mixtures, carminative, and antispasmodic.

DILL: *Anethum graveollens*
    Part used: leaves, seeds
    Use: aromatic, carminative, stomach tonic, colic, sour gassy stomach.

EPAZOTE: *Chenopodium ambrosicides* a plant of the Southwest used in cooking beans
    Part used: leaves

Use: classic seasoning for beans, prevents gas, stimulates milk for nursing mothers, menstrual stimulant, antithelmic.

FENNEL: *Foeniculum vulgare*
Part used: seeds, leaves
Use: stimulant diaphoretic loosens bronchial secretions, emmenagogue, increases secretion of milk, in India used to keep insects away, antispasmotic.

FENUGREEK: *Trigonella foenum-graecum*
Part used: seeds and bulb
Use: preventing fevers, diabetes, inflammations of the stomach and intestines, poultices for abscesses, boils, carbuncles, contains female estrogen, folk remedy for breast enlargement.

GARLIC: *Allium sativum*
Part used: bulb
Use: diaphoretic, diuretic, expectorant, lung disorders, promotes digestion, helps balance blood sugar, expels worms, germicidal, moves blood stagnation and clots, opens vessels, balances blood pressure, protects against heavy metals cadmium and mercury, antioxidant, helps prevent chromosome breakage, increases bile secretion, builds cells, calms nerves, immune stimulant, normalizes calcium metabolism, antibiotic, especially gram negative bacteria.

GINGER: *Zingiber officinale*, Ajenjibre
Part used: root—fresh is best, can be dried and ground
Use: stimulant, carminative, dyspepsia, gas, colic, cramps, nausea, diaphoretic, rubefacient.
CAUTION: do not use if person has gastric ulcers

LAVENDER: *Lavandula officinalis*
Part used: dried flowers
Use: burns, stings, headache, coughs, colds, strong antibacterial action, kills streptococcus, chest infections, sedative, calms anxiety and tension, spasms of digestive tract, nervous headaches; used in massage oil can relax muscles.

MARJORAM: *Organum majorana*
> Part used: leaves
> Use: asthma, indigestion, arthritis, toothache, antioxidant, antifungal.

MUSTARD: *Brassica alba*
> Part used: seeds
> Use: counter irritant, bronchitis, sore throat, stimulant, diuretic, emetic.

NUTMEG: *Myristica fragrans*
> Part used: dried kernel of the seed
> Use: tonic, to flavor medicines, flatulence, nausea and vomiting.

OREGANO: *Origanum vulgare*
> Part used: leaves
> Use: indigestion, tonic, coughs, headache, promotes menses, poultice to soothe painful swollen joints, antiseptic.

OREGANO DE LA SIERRA: *Monarda didyma*
> Part used: flowers, leaves
> A classic Southwest plant grows on mesas when there is rain.
> Use: leaves in cooking, flowers garnish salads, coughs, sore throats, nausea, flatulence, and menstrual cramps.

PARSLEY: *Carum petroselinum*
> Part used; root, seed, leaves
> Use: diuretic, poultice of leaves for bites and stings, high in Vitamin A and C and calcium, arthritis, antispasmodic.

PEPPERCORNS: *Peper nigrum*
> Part used: seeds
> Use: stimulates taste buds, promotes gastric secretions; ground and mixed with honey each morning for excess mucus and sore throats.

PEPPERMINT (any of the mints): *Mentha piperita*
> Part used: leaves and flowers

Use: antispasmodic, nausea, flatulence, diaphoretic, stimulates circulation, heartburn, inhale oil for chest complaints, antiseptic, anesthetic, disinfectant, neuralgic headaches, palpitations of heart, hysteria.

ROSEMARY: *Rosmarinus officinalis*
Part used: leaves, root
Use: tonic, astringent, diaphoretic, stimulant, improves memory, prevention of baldness (nutrition and external), dandruff; stimulates brain and nervous system, depression, headaches.

SAGE: *Salvia officinalis*
Part used: leaves, whole plant
Use: stimulant, astringent, tonic and carminative, stimulates menses, relieves nervous headache, removes mucus from respiratory tract.

SAVORY: *Satureia horrensis*
Part used: leaves
Use: culinary, carminative, colic and gas, first aid for wasp and bee stings.

TARRAGON: *Artemisia dracunculus*
Part used: leaves, root
Use: tonic, induce appetite, root used for toothache.

TEA: *Camellia sinensis*, black or green
Part used: leaves,
Use: green tea is least processed, both types are sources of Vitamin C; antimicrobial, antiinflammatory, astringent, burns, sunburns, gum disease, antioxidant; prevents dental carries, improves beneficial intestinal flora, contains caffeine (30mg to 90mg per cup), stimulant.

THYME: *Thymus vulgaris*
Part used: leaves
Use: antithelmic, antispasmodic, antiseptic, diaphoretic, expectorant, sedative, good for bronchitis, and laryngitis; use

of oil of thyme: contains thymol used in bath as stimulate of circulation, relieves nervous exhaustion.

TURMERIC: *Curcum longa*
Part used: dried rhizome
Use: stimulates flow of bile from liver, stomach disorders, liver ailments, jaundice, increases circulation; antibiotic, anti-inflammatory, improves intestinal flora, blood purifier, promotes proper metabolism in body, tonic to skin; burn powder to keep away mosquitoes.

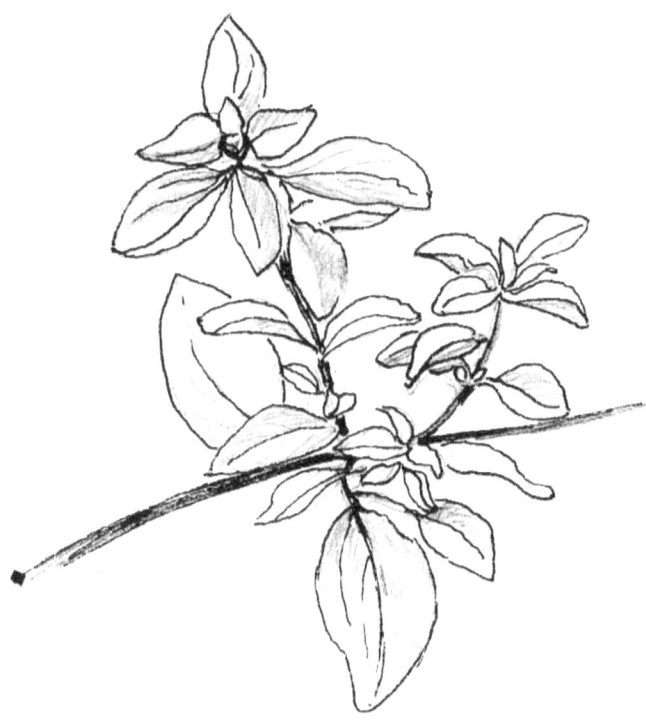

RECIPIES

Rehydration Drink: fluid replacement and electrolyte balance
1 qt. boiled water—water that has been boiled for 10 minutes
½ tsp. table salt
½ tsp baking soda
1 tbl. fructose or 15 tbl. white sugar or 3 tbl. honey or agave syrup
It is wise to keep container full of Rehydration mix, ready for instant use.

Isotonic Eye Wash: Use distilled or boiled water
1 qt. water: 1 tsp salt
1 pt. water: ½ tsp salt
1 c. water: ¼ tsp salt
Salt Free Spice Blends: For your taste buds and your good health:

Herb salt substitute:
Kelp powder: 1/3 cup
Garlic powder: ¼ to 1/3 cup
Onion powder: ¼ to 1/3 cup
Basil powder: ¼ cup
Combine and use in place of salt.

There are many combinations for powdered spices. I have listed a few suggestions. Be creative make up your favorites. Use fresh herbs when possible, dried for future use.

For green vegetables: chives, minced onions, basil, nutmeg, oregano de la sierra (mountain oregano).

For cheese and eggs: dill, chives, parsley, oregano, garlic, and cayenne.

For beans, grains, rice: chilies, cumin, oregano, garlic, mint, parsley, lemon peel, epazote, and mountain oregano.

For fish: dill, lemon juice, grated lemon peel, mustard seed, fennel seed, bay leaf.

For poultry: minced fresh ginger, fresh grated orange peel, sage,

Marinade:

Apple cider vinegar, marjoram, and thyme.
Red meat or vegetarian patties: minced fresh thyme, cloves, grated orange peel, fresh ground black pepper

Herb Vinegar:

These are fun to make using herbs from your kitchen garden. Use apple cider vinegar.
Garlic: 4 cloves, crushed
Chilies: little red-hot ones, 6 dried
Oregano: 4 sprigs of your favorite variety
Place spices in a jar and cover with apple cider vinegar.
Or
Pour off a little of the vinegar, put in the spices, fill to top with the saved vinegar.
Seal containers.
Let set on sunny window seal for two weeks. Change the sprigs for fresh ones, then shake.
It is now ready for use and can be kept for one half to two years.

Bouquet Garni: (a bunch of herbs in a cheese cloth traditionally placed in a stew or soup for flavoring.)

    2 sprigs thyme
    2 sprigs marjoram
    1 bunch parsley stalks
    1 bay leaf

GARGLES:

So useful for colds, sore throat, enlarged tonsils, and post nasal drip.
Combine ¼ tsp of cayenne and sea salt. Add 1 cup hot water.
Sage: make a strong tea; remember, the longer it steeps, the stronger it becomes.

Ginger:

>1 tsp. ginger
>½ cup hot water
>½ squeezed lemon
>1 tsp. honey

Rice Water/Oatmeal Water:

Cook any type rice or oatmeal in twice as much water as usual. Strain the mix. To the liquid add a dash of salt and drink every 4 hours.

Insect Repellent:

1. The easiest way to repel mosquitoes is to add 1 to 2 ounces of citronella oil or lavender to 1 pint of sunflower oil.
2. Make a strong tea (steep 30 minutes) of chamomile or mint, rub on exposed areas.
3. Combine these oils to 1 quart sunflower oil. You now have enough to share with friends.

>1 oz. rue oil
>1 oz. rosemary oil
>1 oz. basil oil
>1 oz. wormwood

Cayenne Liniment

>1 tbl. Cayenne powder
>1 pint apple cider vinegar
>Place in pan and simmer 10 minutes
>Place in previously sterilized bottle

WARNING: Do not place hands anywhere on the body while making this and you may want to wear gloves.

Cayenne Oil:

½ tsp. cayenne powder
1 cup sunflower oil or olive oil
Place the above in a jar and mix well
If you set it in a warm place for two weeks, it will be a stronger remedy.

<u>**WARNING:**</u> *<u>same as above.</u>*

APPENDICES

GLOSSARY

ABRASION: an area on the body where the top layer of skin has been scraped away.

ANALGESIC: Relieves pain

ANESTHETIC: Agent that causes temporary and reversible loss of sensation

ANTHELMINTIC: Kills worms

ANTIBIOTIC: Inhibits growth of bacteria

ANTICOAGULANT: A substance that stops blood from clotting

ANTIOXIDANT: Prevents oxidation or rancidity: A preservative. Antioxidants protect our cells from the effects of free radicals. Free radicals are molecules produced from the breakdown of environmental exposures like: tobacco, cleaning chemicals, substances used in chemotherapy for cancer, pesticides, and radiation. Free radicals can damage cells and researchers think they play a role in heart disease, cancer, and other diseases.

ANTISEPTIC: Prevents or retards growth of bacteria

ANTISPASMODIC: Relieves or prevents spasms, usually of the smooth muscle of the intestinal tract or uterus

ASTRINGENT: Causes constriction of tissues and is used to stop bleeding, secretions, etc.

BITTER: Releases digestive hormones that stimulate the appetite and flow of digestive juices

BOIL: Inflammed pus-filled swelling on the skin

BPA, Bisphenol A: an organic compound used to make polycarbonate plastic and epoxy resins. It is known to be estrogenic. There are concerns regarding exposure of fetuses, infants, and young children. In September 2010 Canada became the first country to declare BPA a toxic substance. It is banned in baby bottles.

BRONCHIAL DILATOR: Something that opens the bronchial passages and allows more oxygen to enter.

CARBUNCLE: A severe abscess or multiple boils in the skin. Typically infected with staphylococcus bacteria.

CARMINATIVE: Relieves and removes gas from intestinal tract

CHOP: Quick heavy strokes using a knife or other sharp tool to cut food into irregular bite-sized pieces.

COLIC: Severe stomach cramps

COMPRESS: External application of herbs that is used to treat superficial ailments, stimulate circulation of blood or lymph, relieve colic, muscle spasms, reduce inflammation, reduce fevers

CONTRACTURE: A condition of shortening and hardening of muscles, tendons or other tissues often leading to deformity and rigidity of joints

COUNTERIRRITANT/RUBAFACIENT: Induces superficial irritation to relieve another irritation or to stimulate circulation

DEMULCENT: Soothes and softens

DECOCTION: A tea that is boiled slowly for 15 to 20 minutes, usually of roots, bark, or large seeds

DIALYSIS: Mechanical purification of blood as a substitute for the normal function of the kidney

DIAPHORETIC: Promotes sweating

DICE: To cut food into small uniform pieces (cubes)

DIURETIC: Increases flow of urine

DOUBLE BOILER: A way of cooking without direct heat. A bottom saucepan is filled with water and the top pan with the mixture to be cooked

DYSPEPSIA: Upset stomach, heartburn

EMETIC: Promotes vomiting

EMMENAGOGUE: Stimulates menstrual flow

EMOLLIENT: Soothes and softens

EXPECTORANT: Stimulates the removal of mucus from lungs

FERMENTATION: The conversion of sugars into alcohols or acids using yeast, bacteria, or both. This process is used for making certain beverages such as: cider, mead, beer, and wine, and to preserve foods: sauerkraut, kimchi, yogurt, or vinegar.

FLATULENCE: Expelled gas from the colon

GANGRENE: Localized death and decomposition of body tissue, resulting from either obstructed circulation or bacterial infection.

GARGLE: The process in which one bubbles a liquid in the mouth as the head tilts backward, goes to the upper part of the throat. It is used for: cleaning the throat, soothing irritated and inflamed mucus membranes, removes bacteria from the throat.

GMO: Genetically modified organisms

GRATE: To cut into very small pieces using a grater

HAEMOSTATIC: Stops internal or external bleeding

INFECTION: The colonization of a host organism by a pathogen. The infecting organism interferes with the normal functioning of the host, can lead to death.

INFLAMMATION: The body's natural response to infections, damaged cells, or irritants. The body tries to remove the injurious stimuli and to initiate the healing process. Inflammation is not the same as infection.

INFUSION: A method of brewing tea, in which boiling water is poured over a plant, leaves, or flowers.

KETOACIDOSIS: A complication of diabetes that occurs when the body cannot use sugar as a fuel and fat is used instead. The by-products of fat breakdown are called ketones and build up in the body. Ketones are poisonous. Warning signs: deep rapid breathing, dry skin, and mouth, flushed face, fruity breathe, nausea and vomiting, stomach pain. The treatment is to correct the high blood sugar levels. Untreated ketoacidosis can lead to severe illness or death.

LAXATIVE: Relieves constipation

MASH: To crush, beat or squeeze a food into a soft state

NERVINE: Stops nervousness and irritability

NETI POT: A device used for irrigating the nasal passages. It can be made of ceramic, glass, metal, or plastic. Typically it has a spout attached near the bottom, often with a handle on the opposite side.

OINTMENT/SALVE: Semi-solid preparations made from beeswax and oil and organic herbal material that are applied to the skin.

PALPITATIONS: Abnormality of heart beat that causes awareness of its beating

POULTICE: A warm moist mass of powdered herbs that is applied directly to the skin in order to: relieve inflammation, draw out poison from venomous bites and stings, skin eruptions, promote proper cleansing and healing of affected area.

PUREE: To puree is to make a smooth creamy substance of liquidized or crushed fruit or vegetables

RUBAFACIENT: A counterirritant: induces superficial irritation to relieve another irritation; stimulates circulation to an area.

SEDATIVE: Sleep inductive

SIMMER: To cook a liquid at just below the boiling point

STEAM INHALATION: Inhalation of warm moist air into the mucus membranes of the respiratory tract.

STEEP: Soak in water or other liquid so as to extract its flavor or to soften it. To soak or saturate (cloth) in water or other liquid.

STERILIZE: Make something free from bacteria or other living microorganisms

STRAIN: To separate liquids from solids by passing through a sieve or cheesecloth

TINCTURE: Alcohol concentration of a plant, an extract.

URIC ACID: An almost insoluble compound, which is a breakdown product of nitrogenous metabolism.

KITCHEN EQUIPMENT

Use only wooden, glass, enamel, or stainless steel equipment. Do not use aluminum. Constituents from some plants can react to form aluminum compounds. Aluminum can leech into the liquids of foods being cooked. Acidic foods cooked in aluminum produce a chloride poison, and neutralizes the digestive juices, making them less acidic, and therefore reducing digestion in the stomach. Unwanted aluminum is deposited in the brain and nervous system, and it will continue to accumulate there. Accumulation of aluminum salts in the brain has been implicated in seizures and reduced mental faculties, and autopsies have found that the brains of Alzheimer's victims have four times the normal amounts of aluminum. Why take chances?

You probably have many of these items already. Do not be overwhelmed. You can start with the very basic. Let your interest be your guide.

1. Measuring cups and spoons
2. Wooden Spoons: Used for stirring and mixing, including a slotted spoon
3. Spatulas
4. Sharp knives: Both smooth and serrated for chopping, paring or cutting
5. Knife sharpener: Nothing can cause more problems in a kitchen than a dull knife.
6. Cutting boards (use wooden only): It is nice to have two, one for garlic and onions and one for everything else. Clean well after using, pouring vinegar over the boards will kill bacteria.
7. Garlic press, not absolutely necessary, but a great tool to get all the juices.
8. Grater, with many sides or attachments, for different foods
9. Spice, seed, and coffee grinder: This may be electric or manual or mortar and pestle.
10. Kitchen thermometer, used to measure temperature of liquids and poultices so they will not burn skin.
11. Stainless steel or enamel pots and pans of various sizes. A double boiler is used when making salves.
12. Strainers: Sieve, and colander

Medicine from the Kitchen

13. Tea balls, (or small strainer): Used for making fresh tea or loose dried tea.
14. Vegetable scrub brush: Used for cleaning produce.
15. Wire whisk
16. Juicer: Used to make fresh vegetable and fruit juices. (This is a major investment; research this and talk with people who own and use juicers.)
17. Hot pads and heat absorbent pads.

OTHER KITCHEN NECESSITIES

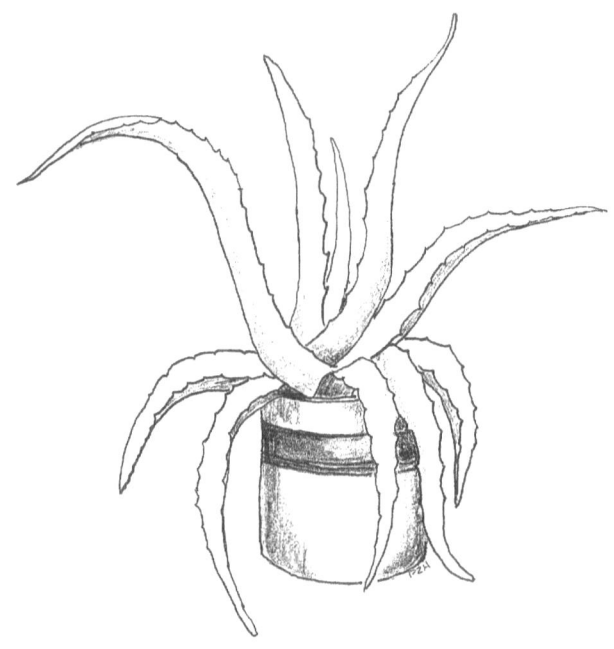

ALOE VERA: *Aloe barbadensis*
>Part used: leaves
>Use: antibacterial heals burns and cuts. The juice soothes and heals an irritated digestive tract. Laxative use of aloe not recommended.

Apple Cider Vinegar

Apple cider vinegar (ACV) is made by crushing fresh organic apples and allowing them to ferment in wooden barrels. When it is mature, it contains a dark cloudy foam called "Mother." Vinegars that contain "Mother" have enzymes and minerals that other vinegars have lost due to over processing and overheating. ACV contains these minerals and trace elements: potassium, calcium, magnesium, phosphorous, chlorine, sodium, sulfur, copper, iron, silicon, and fluorine; these are all vital for a healthy balanced body. My father drank apple cider vinegar, honey, and water daily upon rising. He was a healthy man who rarely had a cold.

Apple cider vinegar contains 55% acetic acid, which gives a ph of 5-7, and this makes it an effective disinfectant agent.

These are a few of the circumstances that have benefited from taking ACV:

- Reduce sinus infections and sore throats
- Cure skin conditions such as acne
- Strengthen the immune system
- Improve digestion
- Increase metabolism
- Prevent kidney stones and urinary tract infections
- Help lower cholesterol
- Help balance blood sugar

As with everything, there are precautions:

- I do not recommend taking vinegar tablets or capsules, these are very concentrated, and if lodged on throat or esophagus can cause damage to the tissues.
- Always dilute any acid drink, taking them "straight" on a long-term basis can erode teeth enamel, giving them a yellowish look and making them more sensitive to heat and cold.
- Moderation: The key to taking any vitamin or mineral, supplement, food, or herbal product is moderation.
- If you are allergic to apples—do not take apple cider vinegar.

I always have one day of the week when I take NO vitamins or supplements, giving the liver a break. One of the many jobs of the liver is breaking down everything that comes into our body into a usable or an excretable form. I may take ACV for several months then switch to water and chlorophyll or only drink aloe vera juice for a few months.

Baking Soda

Sodium bicarbonate or sodium hydrogen carbonate is the chemical compound with the formula $NaHCO2$. It is a white crystalline powder that has a slight alkaline taste. The natural mineral form is known as nahcolite. It is also produced artificially. One of its values is its acid-neutralizing properties. It is used in cooking where it reacts with other components to release carbon dioxide as in helping dough to rise. A paste of baking soda and water can be an effective cleaning and scrubbing agent. Kept in the kitchen it can be used to smother a small fire. Its medicinal uses include: antacid to treat acid indigestion and heartburn. It can treat cases of acidosis and taken in a warm bath it can reduce itching. A paste placed on an insect sting will help draw the poison out.

Honey

Honey is a mixture of monosaccharide sugars and other compounds, such as digestive enzymes and compounds thought to function as antioxidants. Honey contains trace amounts of B Vitamins, folate, Vitamin C, and the minerals: calcium, iron, magnesium, phosphorus, potassium, sodium, and zinc. Each batch of honey is different, depending on the flowers the bees visit.

Things to know when buying, storing, and using honey:

1. Fresh honey flows from a knife in a straight flow.
2. If honey is transparent it has likely been heated and has lost most of its value.
3. Types: Best if certified **organic**.
    a. Comb honey: Honey sold still in the original comb.
    b. Raw honey: Extracted in temperatures under 120 degrees. May contain some pollen and pieces of wax.
    c. Strained: Honey is passed thru a mesh material to remove particles.
4. Storage:
    a. Store in the dark, direct sunlight can destroy enzymes.
    b. Store in a dry area as honey can absorb moisture and might start fermenting or molding.
    c. Three years is the maximum it can be stored.
    d. Use glass or ceramic containers to avoid absorption of heavy metals.
    e. Heating to 98.6 degrees causes it to lose its nutritive value and antimicrobial qualities.

5. PRECAUTION: Not for children under one year. Their underdeveloped digestive systems cannot handle the natural presence of botulism endospores.
6. Do not microwave honey; it reduces enzyme activity and nutritive content—although it does give it a longer shelf life.

Honey has been shown to be a cough suppressant, immune system booster, and free radical cleanser. Research indicates that it promotes blood sugar control and heightens insulin sensitivity. With its low water content, acidic properties (PH 3.2-4.5), and its diluted hydrogen peroxide content, it kills infection-causing organisms. It is especially effective against staphylococcus aurous, which has become a danger to hospitals and now local communities in its mutated form known as methylin resistant staphylococcus aurous, or MRSA.

Olive Oil

From the seeds of the olive tree, *Olea europaea. They* are pressed to make olive oil. Olive oil is a source of Vitamin E, trace elements, and monounsaturated fats. It is nourishing, and also a demulcent, lubricant, laxative; it is moistening, promotes digestion, healing of wounds, and is calming. Extra virgin oil is the least processed.

Salt

Sodium and chloride ions are the two major components of salt. Salt is essential for all human and animal life. When our ancient ancestors left the sea to live on land, they took some of the sea with them enclosed in their bodies. We are actually an inland sea. Salt flavor is one of our basic tastes.

Salt plays an intricate role in regulating the water content for our bodies. Too much or too little can tip the scale and create an imbalance that can lead to death. A deficiency produces muscle cramps, dizziness, and fatal neurological problems.

Excessive intake has been linked to: asthma, edema, heartburn, osteoporosis, duodenal ulcers, gastric ulcers, gastric cancer, high blood pressure, cardiac enlargement, and cardio vascular disease.

Forms of salt

1. Unrefined sea salt: contains trace minerals, but little iodine, tastes slightly bitter.
2. Refined salt: the refining process removes most other minerals out.
3. Table salt: 99% sodium chloride and 1% anti-caking agents, to make it free flowing. Often sodium aluminosilicate and alumino-calcium silicate are used—check your labels carefully
4. Iodized salt: Helps reduce the chance of iodine deficiency. If using sea salt, you must add kelp powder to the salt, include kelp in your diet, or take kelp supplements. Most commercial sea salt comes with iodine added.

Sunflower Oil

The sunflower, *Helianthus annuus*, is a native of Mexico and Peru. Sunflower seeds are a great source of the essential fatty acids necessary for the production of prostaglandins, the hormone-like compounds that regulate every function in the body at the molecular level. It is high in linoleic and oleic acids and is a combination of mono-unsaturated and polyunsaturated fats with a low saturated fat level. It is high in Vitamin E, lecithin and carotenoids. There are many healthful reasons to use sunflower oil. It has been shown to have cholesterol-reducing properties. Vitamin E is an antioxidant that protects the heart. Research has shown that linoleic and linolenic acids are beneficial in diabetes. The oil helps the skin retain moisture and provides a protective barrier that resists infection. It is very soothing to the skin. The seeds are diuretic and have expectorant properties. It has been used in the treatment of bronchial, laryngeal, and other pulmonary conditions, colds, and coughs. It is my favorite and my kitchen always has a ready supply

Water

Everything originated in water. Everything will be sustained by water. Johann Wolfgang Goethe, German philosopher and poet

Water sustains all life on Earth, and Earth is the only planet in our universe that has liquid water on its surface. Two thirds or 70%

of our body's total weight is water. Our body is designed to run on water. We function more efficiently when we are properly hydrated. Eight, eight ounce glasses of water (½ Gallon) are the minimal amount to drink per day. This varies with activity, climate, and season. The proper amount of water can prevent headaches, keep blood pressure from going dangerously low (blood pressure varies with blood volume), aids digestion, helps kidneys with their work of regulating body fluid balance; with too much water loss the blood flow to the brain decreases, causing headache, nausea, confusion, and eventual collapse. Even mild dehydration slows down metabolism as much as 3%. Want to lose weight? Drink water. Lack of water is the number one cause of daytime fatigue. Having trouble focusing on the computer screen or reading a printed page? Cannot do basic math? Memory a bit fuzzy? How much water did you drink today? Even a 2% drop in body water can cause these symptoms. So, relax, sit in your favorite chair, and enjoy a nice cool refreshing glass of pure, uncontaminated water.

U.S. AND METRIC MEASURES

½ teaspoon = 30 drops
1 teaspoon = 60 drops = 5 milliliters
3 teaspoons = 1 tablespoon = 1/2 fluid ounce
2 tablespoons = 1 fl. ounce
4 tablespoons = ¼ cup = 2 fl. ounces
8 tablespoons = ½ cup = 4 fl ounces
16 tablespoons = 1 cup = 8 fl. ounces
2 cups = 1 pint = 16 fl. ounces
  = ½ liter
4 cups = 1 quart = 2 pints = 1 liter
4 quarts = 1 gallon = 3.7 liters
16 ounces dry = 1 pound

Measuring dry herbs:

The best way to measure out ounces is with a simple pan balance scale. These can be purchased from scientific supply stores and some drugstores. Kitchen scales are available for under twenty dollars. Postage scales may also be used.

Measuring temperatures:

FAHRENHEIT (at sea level) CELSIUS/CENTIGRADE

32 degrees F water freezes = 0 degrees C
115 degrees F water simmers = 46 degrees C
130 degrees F water scalds = 54 degrees C
212 degrees F water boils = 100 degrees C

BASIC FIRST AID KITS

Basic first aid kits for home, car, camping, and hiking can be purchased or assembled by the individual or family. A good first aid book is essential (such as the one by the American Red Cross).

When selecting or making kits, keep this in mind:

1. Kit should be large enough.
2. Arrange contents so items can be found quickly.
3. Keep all medicine out of reach of children.
4. Excessive sun/heat will deteriorate both pharmaceuticals and botanicals.
5. Check the contents every few months for outdated or damaged supplies.

BASIC SUPPLIES

- First aid book
- Band-aids, assorted sizes
- Non stick dressings, assorted sizes
- Butterfly bandages or steri-strips, assorted sizes
- Gauze pads, 2 x 2" or 4 x 4" sizes
- Sterile eye patches
- Roller gauze, 2" and 4"
- Elastic wrap (ace bandages) 2" and 4"
- Triangular bandages
- Adhesive tape
- Bandage compresses (ABD pads)
- Cotton swabs
- Cotton balls
- Safety pins
- Steel sewing needles
- Paper clips
- Scissors
- Tweezers
- Soap
- Matches
- Snakebite kit

- Thermometer: Replace all mercury thermometers. Take to household hazardous waste at the solid waste landfill. Use ear or temporal scanner thermometers.
- Alcohol and peroxide
- Gloves
- Baggies to hold blood and infectious waste

OTHER HELPFUL ADDITIONS TO FIRST AID KIT

- Syrup of Ipecac: a botanical extract from the *Cephaelis ipecacuanha* plant of South America. It is a natural irritant to the stomach that safely induces vomiting in 20 minutes.
- Olbas oil: an all purpose oil that soothes insect stings, muscle soreness, burns, and sun burn, from the essential oils of:
    Eucalyptus
    Peppermint
    Cajuput
    Juniper
    Wintergreen
- Rescue Remedy: A Bach flower remedy for cases of shock, panic, and stress.
- Arnica: homeopathic pills and salve: to reduce swelling from injuries.

HOME MEDICAL WASTE DISPOSAL

Use gloves when cleaning or disposing of materials that contain blood or possible infectious matter. Wash your hands before and after using the gloves. Use a heavy duty plastic bag that has a biohazard label. You may copy and paste the label on the waste bag.

If a person has a diagnosed infectious disease and is at home, consult the state health department for instructions that comply with your state's regulations.

RESOURCES AND REFERENCES

- American Academy of Orthopedic Surgeons, http://www.aaos.org
- Auerbach, Paul MD *Medicine for the Outdoors* 1986, Little, Brown, and Company
- Bigfoot, Peter; Zella, Angelique, *Venomous Bites and Stings; Natural Remedies* 1980 Peter Bigfoot
- Buchman, Dian *Herbal Medicine* 1980 Gramercy Publishing Company
- Cordes, Betty CRNA *Pocket Guide to Emergency First Aid* 2005 A Pocket guides Publishing Book
- Forgey, William MD *Wilderness Medicine* 1987 ICS Books, Inc.
- *Herbal Medicine: Expanded Commission E Monographs* 2000 Integrative Medicine Communications
- IDEA Health and Fitness Association http://www.ideafit.com/fitness.com/fallprevention-program
- Jarvis, D.C. MD *Folk Medicine* 1958 Fawcett Publications
- Kloss, Jethro *Back to Eden* 1971 Lancer Books
- Moore, Michael S. *Medicinal Plants of the Mountain West* 1979 Museum of New Mexico Press, Notes from classes and personal communication
- *PDR for Herbal Medicine* 4th edition 2007 Thomas Healthcare Inc.
- *Rodale's Illustrated Encyclopedia of Herbs* 1987 Rodale Press
- *Survival Wisdom and Know-how* 2007 Black Dog and Leventhal Publishers
- Tso, Sam Dineh healer, personal communication
- Werner, David *Where There Is No Doctor* 1977 Hesperian Foundation
- Wilderness Medicine Conference, Santa Fe, New Mexico 2011
- Wilkerson, James MD *Medicine for Mountaineering 3rd Edition* The Mountaineers
- Whitefeather, Willy, personal communication

FAMILY MEDICAL INFORMATION

NAME _____
AGE _____ BLOOD TYPE _____
ALLERGIES AND REACTIONS
_____
_____
_____

OTHER MEDICAL INFORMATION: PREVIOUS ILLNESSES AND OPERATIONS, INJURIES, INSECT OR ANIMAL BITES REQUIRING MEDICAL ATTENTION, FAMILY HISTORY, AND RECENT EXPOSURES TO INFECTIONS
_____
_____
_____
_____
_____

MEDICATIONS, VITAMINS, SUPPLEMENTS, HERBAL PRODUCTS TAKEN ON A DAILY BASIS, INCLUDE DOSAGES, THIS IS ESPECIALLY IMPORTANT IF TAKING INSULIN OR DIABETIC MEDICATIONS
_____
_____
_____
_____
_____

DATE LAST TETANUS SHOT OR BOOSTER _____

YOUR SPACE

THIS IS "YOUR" SPACE TO RECORD: DATE INCIDENT OCCURRED, TO WHOM DID IT OCCUR, REMEDIES USED, OUTCOMES, WHAT WORKED/DID NOT WORK.

_____
_____
_____
_____
_____
_____
_____
_____
_____
_____
_____
_____
_____
_____
_____
_____
_____
_____
_____
_____
_____
_____
_____
_____
_____
_____
_____
_____
_____
_____
_____

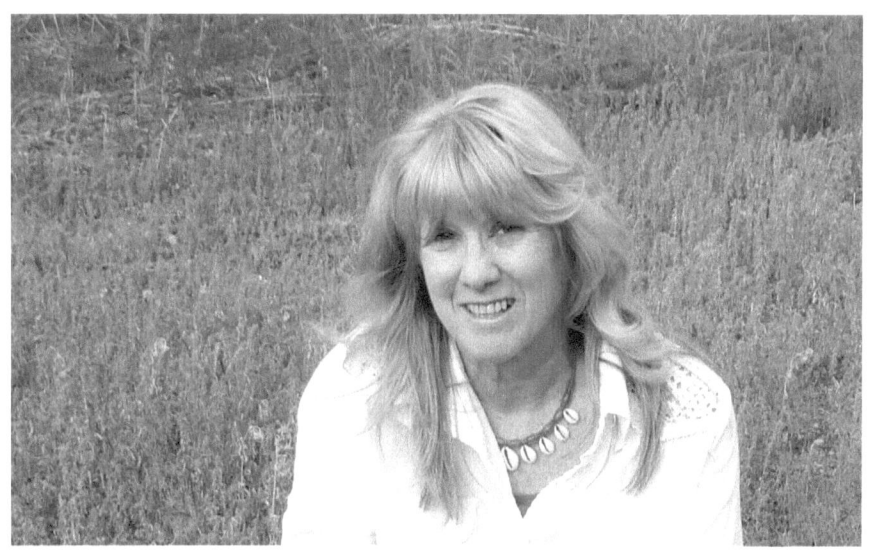

About Jessie Emerson

- Registered nurse since 1965
- Graduate Santa Fe School of Natural Medicine, 1979
- Certified Clinical Herbalist, Graduate Michael S. Moore's Southwest School of Botanical Medicine, Silver City, New Mexico, 1989
- Graduate Prescott College, "Sustainable Community Development", 2004
- Ecovillage Design Program, Gaia Education, Findhorn, Scotland, 2007
- Ongoing cross-culture education and training with Native American healers and herbalists
- Over 30 years practice as an alternative healthcare professional
- Producer, director, and writer of the educational documentary on Diabetes, "Like the Moosni Turtle, the Comcaac will Endure"; and "Just an Old Fashioned Herbalist", the story of Southwest herbalist, Michael S. Moore.
- Owner of Oso Productions and Oso Herbals

Emerson says: "Our goal is to collect and share information to educate and empower people to reconnect and heal Mother Earth, communities, and ourselves . . . . We do this by promoting sustainability principles, and I engage in this by using my skills, knowledge, and experiences as a nurse and clinical herbalist to promote wellness and prevent disease, and by working in collaboration with those groups and individuals who desire to prevent further damage to Gaia—people who want to help bring the Earth and themselves back into balance."

When Jessie and her dog Sophie aren't in the mountains or deserts, they may be found in the garden. Jessie teaches wild food identification and cooking, and she is often in her kitchen, but Sophie only goes in by invitation. You can attend her classes in, "Medicine from the Kitchen," and "Herbal Medicine in the Wilds." Other services, healing programs, and educational programs she offers:

Body systems regulation and tonification; Immune system enhancement; Body detoxification of free radicals from environmental pollutants; Chemo and radiation therapies; Liver cleansing and strengthening; Recuperation after hospitalization; Customized herbal medicine chests and first aid kits; Creating your own medicinal garden, from the soil up; Basic Herbology, including salve and tincture preparations; Herbology for health care professionals; Diabetic education, "The Natural Approach to Diabetes"; Field work in plant identification and plant meditation.

Contact Jessie at osoherbalsjessie@gmail.com or P.O. Box 605, Alcalde, New Mexico 87511

www.ingramcontent.com/pod-product-compliance
Lightning Source LLC
Chambersburg PA
CBHW030911180526
45163CB00004B/1790